Lung Screening: Updates and Access

Editors

KEI SUZUKI
DUYKHANH P. CEPPA

THORACIC SURGERY CLINICS

www.thoracic.theclinics.com

Consulting Editor
VIRGINIA R. LITLE

November 2023 • Volume 33 • Number 4

ELSEVIER

1600 John F. Kennedy Boulevard • Suite 1800 • Philadelphia, Pennsylvania, 19103-2899

http://www.thoracic.theclinics.com

THORACIC SURGERY CLINICS Volume 33, Number 4
November 2023 ISSN 1547-4127, ISBN-13: 978-0-443-18336-2

Editor: John Vassallo (j.vassallo@elsevier.com)
Developmental Editor: Jessica Nicole B. Cañaberal

Thoracic Surgery Clinics (ISSN 1547-4127) is published quarterly by Elsevier Inc., 360 Park Avenue South, New York, NY 10010-1710. Months of publication are February, May, August, and November. Business and editorial offices: 1600 John F. Kennedy Boulevard, Suite 1800, Philadelphia, PA 19103-2899. Periodicals postage paid at New York, NY, and additional mailing offices. Subscription prices are $417.00 per year (US individuals), $681.00 per year (US institutions), $100.00 per year (US students), $487.00 per year (Canadian individuals), $881.00 per year (Canadian institutions), $100.00 per year (Canadian students), $225.00 per year (international students), $509.00 per year (international individuals), and $881.00 per year (international institutions). Foreign air speed delivery is included in all Clinics' subscription prices. All prices are subject to change without notice. **POSTMASTER:** Send address changes to Thoracic Surgery Clinics, Elsevier Health Sciences Division, Subscription Customer Service, 3251 Riverport Lane, Maryland Heights, MO 63043. **Customer Service (orders, claims, online, change of address): Telephone: 1-800-654-2452 (U.S. and Canada); 314-447-8871 (outside U.S. and Canada). Fax: 314-447-8029. E-mail: journalscustomerservice-usa@elsevier.com (for print support); journalsonlinesupport-usa@elsevier.com (for online support).**

Reprints. For copies of 100 or more, of articles in this publication, please contact Commercial Rights Department, Elsevier Inc., 360 Park Avenue South, New York, NY 10010-1710. Tel: 212-633-3874; Fax: 212-633-3820; E-mail: reprints@elsevier.com.

Thoracic Surgery Clinics is covered in *MEDLINE/PubMed (Index Medicus), EMBASE/Excerpta Medica, Science Citation Index Expanded (SciSearch®), Journal Citation Reports/Science Edition,* and *Current Contents®/Clinical Medicine.*

Contributors

CONSULTING EDITOR

VIRGINIA R. LITLE, MD
Chief of Thoracic Surgery, Division of Thoracic Surgery, Department of Surgery, St.
Elizabeth's Medical Center, Brighton, Massachusetts, USA

EDITORS

DUYKHANH P. CEPPA, MD
Associate Professor of Surgery, Indiana University School of Medicine, Program Director, Cardiothoracic Surgery Residency, Deputy Chief of Surgery, Roudebush VA Medical Center, Indianapolis, Indiana, USA

KEI SUZUKI, MD, MS, FACS
Director of Thoracic Surgery Research, Schar Cancer Institute, Inova Health Systems, Assistant Professor, University of Virginia School of Medicine, Fairfax, Virginia, USA

AUTHORS

SCOTT J. ADAMS, MD, PhD
Department of Radiology, Stanford University School of Medicine, Stanford, California, USA

MARA B. ANTONOFF, MD
Department of Thoracic and Cardiovascular Surgery, The University of Texas MD Anderson Cancer Center, Houston, Texas, USA

REGINA BARZILAY, PhD
Department of Electrical Engineering and Computer Science, Jameel Clinic, Massachusetts Institute of Technology, Cambridge, Massachusetts, USA

CONNOR J. BRIDGES, BS
Geisel School of Medicine, Hanover, New Hampshire, USA

ALEJANDRA CARDONA-DEL VALLE, MD
Department of Radiology, University of Puerto Rico School of Medicine, San Juan, Puerto Rico

RUTH C. CARLOS, MD, MS
Department of Radiology, University of Michigan, Ann Arbor, Michigan, USA

LISA CARTER-BAWA, PHD, APRN, ANP-C, FAAN
Director, Cancer Prevention Precision Control Institute, Center for Discovery and Innovation, Professor of Medical Sciences, Hackensack Meridian School of Medicine, Hackensack Meridian Health, Nutley, New Jersey, USA

NEEL P. CHUDGAR, MD
Assistant Professor of Cardiovascular and Thoracic Surgery, Montefiore Medical Center at the Albert Einstein College of Medicine, Bronx, New York, USA

RICHARD J. CURLEY, DrPH
Department of Surgery, City of Hope Comprehensive Cancer Center, Duarte, California, USA

NATHANIEL DEBOEVER, MD
Department of Thoracic and Cardiovascular Surgery, The University of Texas MD Anderson Cancer Center, Houston, Texas, USA

LORETTA ERHUNMWUNSEE, MD, FACS
Departments of Surgery and Population Sciences, City of Hope Comprehensive Cancer Center, Duarte, California, USA

FLORIAN J. FINTELMANN, MD
Harvard Medical School, Department of
Radiology, Massachusetts General Hospital,
Boston, Massachusetts, USA

EFREN J. FLORES, MD
Division of Thoracic Imaging, Department of
Radiology, Massachusetts General Hospital,
Boston, Massachusetts, USA

ZACHARY HARTLEY-BLOSSOM, MD, MBA
Division of Thoracic Imaging, Department of
Radiology, Massachusetts General Hospital,
Boston, Massachusetts, USA

RIAN M. HASSON, MD, FACS
Department of Surgery, Section of Thoracic
Surgery, Dartmouth-Hitchcock Medical
Center, The Dartmouth Institute of Health
Policy and Clinical Practice, Lebanon, New
Hampshire, USA; Geisel School of Medicine,
Hanover, New Hampshire, USA

CHI-FU JEFFREY YANG, MD
Assistant Professor of Surgery, Division of
Thoracic Surgery, Massachusetts General
Hospital, Boston, Massachusetts, USA

MADISON R. KOCHER, MD, MBA
Clinical Associate of Radiology, Division of
Cardiothoracic Imaging, Department of
Radiology, Duke University School of
Medicine, Durham, North Carolina, USA

SANGKAVI KUHAN, BS
Research Assistant, Division of Thoracic
Surgery, Massachusetts General Hospital,
Boston, Massachusetts, USA

KATHERINE T. LEOPOLD, BS
Hackensack University School of Medicine,
Nutley, New Jersey, USA

PETER MIKHAEL, BSc
Department of Electrical Engineering and
Computer Science, Jameel Clinic,
Massachusetts Institute of Technology,
Cambridge, Massachusetts, USA

TAKAHIRO MIMAE, MD, PhD
Department of Surgical Oncology, Hiroshima
University, Hiroshima, Japan

CLAUDIA MUNS-APONTE, BS
Department of Radiology, University of Puerto
Rico School of Medicine, San Juan, Puerto
Rico

PIERGIORGIO MURIANA, MD
Department of Thoracic Surgery, San Raffaele
Scientific Institute, Milan, Italy

PIERLUIGI NOVELLIS, MD
Department of Thoracic Surgery, San Raffaele
Scientific Institute, Milan, Italy

MORIHITO OKADA, MD, PhD
Department of Surgical Oncology, Hiroshima
University, Hiroshima, Japan

EDWIN J. OSTRIN, MD, PhD
Department of General Internal Medicine,
Pulmonary Medicine, The University of Texas
MD Anderson Cancer Center, Houston, Texas,
USA

ALEXANDRA L. POTTER, BS
Research Assistant, Division of Thoracic
Surgery, Massachusetts General Hospital,
Boston, Massachusetts, USA

FRANCESCA ROSSETTI, MD
Department of Thoracic Surgery, San Raffaele
Scientific Institute, Milan, Italy

LORI C. SAKODA, PhD, MPH
Research Scientist, Division of Research,
Kaiser Permanente Northern California,
Oakland, California, USA

HAI V.N. SALFITY, MD, MPH
Assistant Professor of Surgery, Division of
Thoracic Surgery, Department of Surgery,
University of Cincinnati School of Medicine,
Cincinnati, Ohio, USA

PRIYANKA SENTHIL, BS
Research Assistant, Division of Thoracic
Surgery, Massachusetts General Hospital,
Boston, Massachusetts, USA

LECIA V. SEQUIST, MD, MPH
Department of Medicine, Massachusetts
General Hospital, Harvard Medical School,
Boston, Massachusetts, USA

BRENDON M. STILES, MD
Chief, Division of Thoracic Surgery and
Surgical Oncology, Professor of
Cardiovascular and Thoracic Surgery,
Montefiore Medical Center at the Albert
Einstein College of Medicine

CYNTHIA J. SUSAI, MD
Resident Physician, UCSF East Bay General
Surgery, Oakland, California, USA

TINA D. TAILOR, MD
Associate Professor of Radiology, Division of
Cardiothoracic Imaging, Department of
Radiology, Duke University School of
Medicine, Durham, North Carolina, USA

BETTY C. TONG, MD, MHS, MS
Associate Professor of Surgery, Division of
Thoracic Surgery, Department of Surgery,
Duke University School of Medicine, Durham,
North Carolina, USA

NEHA UDAYAKUMAR, MD
Department of Radiology, Massachusetts
General Hospital, Boston, Massachusetts,
USA

JEFFREY B. VELOTTA, MD
Thoracic Surgeon, Department of Thoracic
Surgery, Kaiser Permanente Northern
California, Oakland, California,
USA

GIULIA VERONESI, MD
Department of Thoracic Surgery, San Raffaele
Scientific Institute, School of Medicine and
Surgery, Vita-Salute San Raffaele University,
Milan, Italy

JEREMY WOHLWEND, ME
Department of Electrical Engineering and
Computer Science, Jameel Clinic,
Massachusetts Institute of Technology,
Cambridge, Massachusetts, USA

Contents

> Lung cancer represents a large burden on society with a staggering incidence and mortality rate that has steadily increased until recently. The impetus to design an effective screening program for the deadliest cancer in the United States and worldwide began in 1950. It has taken more than 50 years of numerous clinical trials and continued persistence to arrive at the development of modern-day screening program. As the program continues to grow, it is important for clinicians to understand its evolution, track outcomes, and continually assess the impact and bias of screening on the medical, social, and economic systems.

> Lung cancer screening has been shown to reduce lung cancer mortality and is recommended for individuals meeting age and smoking history criteria. Despite the expansion of lung cancer screening guidelines in 2021, racial/ethnic and sex disparities persist. High-risk racial minorities and women are more likely to be diagnosed with lung cancer at younger ages and have lower smoking histories when compared with White and male counterparts, resulting in higher rates of ineligibility for screening. Risk prediction models, biomarkers, and deep learning may help refine the selection of individuals who would benefit from screening.

> Lung cancer screening improves lung-cancer specific and potentially overall survival; however, uptake rates are concerningly low. Several barriers to screening exist and require a systemic approach to address. The authors describe their approach toward building a centralized lung cancer screening program at an urban academic center along with lessons learned. To this end, the identification of involved stakeholders, evaluation of community barriers and needs, optimization of the electronic health system, and implementation of system of standardized follow-up for patients are processes for consideration. Perhaps most important to undertaking this endeavor is the need to customize each program and maintain adaptability.

In the context of the Conceptual Model for Lung Cancer Screening Participation, this article describes patient barriers to lung cancer screening highlighting current interventions. Patient barriers include cognitive factors (lack of awareness, limited information/misinformation, and low perceived risk), factors related to access (logistical issues, no provider recommendation, cost, and other financial/social factors), and psychological factors (fear, fatalism, lung cancer worry, and stigma). Current interventions include the use of educational materials/presentations to address cognitive barriers, use of direct outreach and structural change to address factors related to access, and use of educational material focused on psychological barriers to address psychological barriers.

Rural and racial/ethnic minority communities experience higher risk and mortality from lung cancer. Lung cancer screening with low-dose computed tomography reduces mortality. However, disparities persist in the uptake of lung cancer screening, especially in marginalized communities. Barriers to lung cancer screening are multilevel and include patient, provider, and system-level barriers. This discussion highlights the key barriers faced by rural and racial/ethnic minority communities.

Identifying and managing lung cancer, the leading cause of cancer-specific mortality, depend on multiple medical and sociodemographic factors. Humanomics is a model that acknowledges that negative societal stressors from systemic inequity affect individual health by altering pro-inflammatory gene expression. The same factors which may predispose individuals to lung cancer may also obstruct equitably prompt diagnosis and treatment. Increasing lung cancer screening access can lessen disparities in outcomes among disproportionately affected communities. Here, the authors describe several individual, provider, and health system-level obstacles to lung cancer screening and offer actionable solutions to increase access.

Several randomized and observational studies on lung cancer screening held in Europe significantly contributed to the knowledge on low-dose computed tomography screening targets in high-risk individuals with smoking history and older than 50 years. In particular, steps forward have been made in the field of risk modeling, screening interval, diagnostic protocol with volumetry, optimization, overdiagnosis estimation, oncological outcome, oncological risk due to radiation exposure, recruitment, and communication strategy.

Lung cancer is the leading cause of cancer-related mortality in Japan and world-wide. Early detection of lung cancer is an important strategy for decreasing mortality. Advances in diagnostic imaging have made it possible to detect lung cancer at an early stage in medical practice. Conversely, screening of asymptomatic healthy populations is recommended only when the evidence shows the benefits of regular intervention. Due to a variety of evidence and racial differences, screening methods vary from country to country. This article focused on the perspective of lung cancer screening in Japan.

Recent advances in artificial intelligence and machine learning (AI/ML) hold substantial promise to address some of the current challenges in lung cancer screening and improve health equity. This article reviews the status and future directions of AI/ML tools in the lung cancer screening workflow, focusing on determining screening eligibility, radiation dose reduction and image denoising for low-dose chest computed tomography (CT), lung nodule detection, lung nodule classification, and determining optimal screening intervals. AI/ML tools can assess for chronic diseases on CT, which creates opportunities to improve population health through opportunistic screening.

Current lung cancer screening protocols use low-dose computed tomography scans in selected high-risk individuals. Unfortunately, utilization is low, and the rate of false-positive screens is high. Peripheral biomarkers carry meaningful promise in diagnosing and monitoring cancer with added potential advantages reducing invasive procedures and improving turnaround time. Herein, the use of such blood-based assays is considered as an adjunct to further utilization and accuracy of lung cancer screening.

The updated US Preventive Services Task Force guidelines on lung cancer screening have significantly expanded the population of screening eligible adults, among whom the balance of benefits and harms associated with lung cancer screening vary considerably. Clinical adjuncts are additional information and tools that can guide decision-making to optimally screen individuals who are most likely to benefit. Proposed adjuncts include integration of clinical history, risk prediction models, shared-decision-making tools, and biomarker tests at key steps in the screening process. Although evidence regarding their clinical utility and implementation is still evolving, they carry significant promise in optimizing screening effectiveness and efficiency for lung cancer.

THORACIC SURGERY CLINICS

SERIES OF RELATED INTEREST

Advances in Surgery
http://www.advancessurgery.com/

Surgical Clinics
http://www.surgical.theclinics.com/

Surgical Oncology Clinics
https://www.surgonc.theclinics.com/

THE CLINICS ARE AVAILABLE ONLINE!
Access your subscription at:
www.theclinics.com

Foreword
Just the Facts, Ma'am

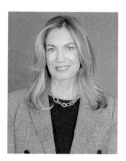

Virginia R. Litle, MD
Consulting Editor

What are some current facts about fear and about cancer screening? (1) It took 50 years for colon and breast cancer screening to become standards of care in preventative medicine, and now more than 60% of eligible folks are screened routinely. People fear cancer. (2) It has taken 50% more time for implementation of lung cancer screening (LCS) with low-dose imaging, and only 6% of eligible people are screened. People fear lung cancer screening because they fear the diagnosis. (3) And on the general topic of fear, Artificial Intelligence (AI) has been generating a lot of it lately. It is the worst of times or is it the best of times? Did I have ChatGPT write this? No. Should I have? Maybe. Let's try to see the bright side here. Lung cancer mortalities are improving, and LCS is a contributing factor along with immunotherapy and targeted therapy. AI and machine learning continue to be investigated to improve interpretation of nodule and malignancy risk as well as to stratify individuals with regards to clinical criteria and imaging. Liquid biopsies are potential future adjuncts to screening. The future direction is bright indeed, and we hope, will have applications for never smokers as well.

As we learn from our contributors in this issue, the side benefits of screening also address other smoking-related illnesses. As Muriana and coauthors describe here, when a risk-prediction tool like the PLCOm2012 model is applied to a subset of folks with a smoking history, they are screened not only for lung cancer but also for COPD and cardiovascular disease—the number one killer in many countries. The broader implications of screening apply to our whole cardiothoracic world.

In this issue of *Thoracic Surgery Clinics*, Guest Editors Drs Mimi Ceppa and Kei Suzuki have collated a thorough range of content to inform us about the current state of lung cancer screening. One big message from multiple submissions in this issue is that we are still missing the boat on addressing inequity in delivery of lung cancer screening to eligible people and that broadening age and smoking history criteria actually widens the gap.

As surgeon/physician/scientists continue to improve screening criteria with biomarker identification, to optimize nodule interpretation with machine learning, and to optimize risk prediction models, we clinicians have actionable items to improve screening rates for eligible people: (1) Educate primary care physicians (PCPs) about screening criteria. (2) Work with community leaders in underscreened areas to connect with eligible folks about the benefits of screening and of continuing with follow-up imaging. (3) Offer a centralized clinic for PCPs and other physicians to send their patients who may be screen eligible or who have incidental nodules. Follow-up adherence rates improve with such programs.

Thank you to Drs Ceppa and Suzuki and to all the socially and forward-thinking contributors of this *Thoracic Surgery Clinics* issue about Lung Cancer Screening. Remember the key to

Thorac Surg Clin 33 (2023) xi–xii
https://doi.org/10.1016/j.thorsurg.2023.06.001
1547-4127/23/© 2023 Published by Elsevier Inc.

improvement is constant evolution, and where we are in LCS is in constant evolution. It is exciting to see the sophisticated advances with machine learning, biomarkers, and risk prediction models; however, we must continue to apply the human learning component as well and educate the gate-keepers, including our primary care colleagues and community folks, who can help reduce the inequity gap in delivery of this significant preventa-tive care advancement in our professional lifetime.

Sincerely,

Virginia R. Litle, MD
Division of Thoracic Surgery
Department of Surgery
St. Elizabeth's Medical Center, 11 Nevins Street
Suite 201
Brighton, MA 02135, USA

E-mail address:
vlitle@gmail.com

Preface

Lung Cancer Screening: Where Are We, and How Can We Improve?

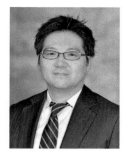
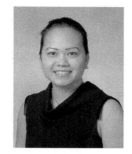

Kei Suzuki, MD   DuyKhanh P. Ceppa, MD
Editors

Since the National Lung Screening Trial demonstrated a 20% decrease in lung cancer mortality in 2011,[1] the eligibility criteria were recently expanded in 2021.[2] While this has increased the population eligible for screening, lung cancer screening rates remain significantly lower compared with other well-established cancer screening rates and remains at a low 5.8% of the eligible population.[3] As we look to improve the lung cancer screening process, we herein review pertinent topics, such as a review of the data supporting screening for lung cancer, building a screening program, increasing screening rates in eligible populations, and how to better target the high-risk population.

In this issue, we first focus on the historical and current state of screening, highlighting the changes we have seen with the recent updates in the 2021 USPSTF guidelines.[3] Salfity and colleagues summarize the historical journey and prudently elaborate the details of imaging fundamentals that allow for accurate assessment of lung nodules. The article on current guidelines by Senthil and colleagues brings to light the shortcomings of the most current guidelines that we must work to address. How to build and grow a successful screening program, especially in safety net settings, is reviewed by Chudgar and colleagues. The authors demonstrate the systemic and multidisciplinary manner in which barriers to screening should be approached in order to build a successful program. Surveying the progress we have made so far in lung cancer screening and overcoming the associated challenges and

controversies inform us on future directions. In order to improve the screening rate, we must first know the specific barriers. We address the multifactorial barriers to screening at different levels, focusing on patient, physician, and system-level factors (access, disparity, humanomics), with potential solutions for each. Leopold and colleagues delve deeply into the patient factors that result in barriers to screening, touching on different subsets of populations and looking at the whole patient by including cognitive and psychological factors, as well as previous attempts at overcoming said barriers. Hartley-Bossom and colleagues explore the lesser-known topic of humanomics and how this can inevitably impact predisposition for cancer and provide potential leads for further research opportunities that could provide answers to closing the gap in disparities in care and outcomes. The highlight on underserved communities and disparities in lung cancer screening that Hasson and colleagues explain so well will hopefully help take further informed steps in reaching these populations. We then gain further insights into the worldwide perspectives in lung cancer screening, with Muriana and colleagues nicely summarizing the European experience and Mimae and colleagues giving us the unique Japanese perspective of screening, especially in the non–high-risk group. Finally, we review potential adjunct tools to improve the yield of screening. The adjunctive clinical prediction models and developing biomarkers are detailed by Susai and colleagues and can provide important directions for overcoming

Thorac Surg Clin 33 (2023) xiii–xiv
https://doi.org/10.1016/j.thorsurg.2023.04.018
1547-4127/23/

the deficits we have with the current screening process. Adams and colleagues focus on the technology of artificial intelligence and machine learning as tools to increase the sensitivity and specificity of screening as well as potentially provide another predictive tool to identify those who would most benefit from screening. Last, Deboever and colleagues elaborate on the current advancements in the liquid biopsy technology and how this could provide a more personalized and synergistic tool to complement our current practices.

We would like to thank all of the authors for being fierce leaders in our field, for tackling the challenging task of increasing the adoption of lung screening, and for their time in documenting their expertise in these excellent articles. We would like to acknowledge the support of John Vassallo and Jessica Cañaberal in facilitating the execution of this special issue. Last, we would like to thank Virginia Litle for the honor and invitation to serve guest editors. We hope you will see that the topics and authors were deliberately selected, and we hope that you enjoy this issue!

Kei Suzuki, MD
Director of Thoracic Surgery Research
Schar Cancer Institute
Inova Health Systems
Assistant Professor
University of Virginia School of Medicine
8081 Innovation Park Drive
Fairfax, VA 22031, USA

DuyKhanh P. Ceppa, MD
Associate Professor of Surgery
Indiana University School of Medicine
Program Director, Cardiothoracic Surgery
Residency
Deputy Chief of Surgery
Roudebush VA Medical Center
545 Barnhill Drive
Indianapolis, IN 46202, USA

E-mail addresses:
Kei.suzuki@inova.org (K. Suzuki)
dpceppa@iupui.edu (D.P. Ceppa)

REFERENCES

1. National Lung Screening Trial Research Team, Aberle DR, Berg CD, Black WC, et al. The National Lung Screening Trial: overview and study design. Radiology 2011;258(1):243–53. https://doi.org/10.1148/radiol.10091808.
2. US Preventive Services Task Force, Krist AH, Davidson KW, Mangione CM, et al. Screening for Lung Cancer: US Preventive Services Task Force Recommendation Statement. JAMA 2021;325(10):962–70. https://doi.org/10.1001/jama.2021.1117.
3. American Lung Association (2022, November). State of lung cancer: Key findings. State of Lung Cancer | Key Findings | American Lung Association. Available at: https://www.lung.org/research/state-of-lung-cancer/key-findings. Accessed April 5, 2023.

Historical Perspective on Lung Cancer Screening

Hai V.N. Salfity, MD, MPH[a],*, Betty C. Tong, MD, MHS, MS[b], Madison R. Kocher, MD, MBA[c],
Tina D. Tailor, MD[c]

KEYWORDS

- Lung cancer screening • Low-dose CT • LDCT • Screening history

KEY POINTS

- Historical efforts for performing lung cancer screening with chest radiography and sputum cytology were not sensitive enough to detect early-stage cancer or yield a mortality benefit.
- Low-dose computed tomography (LDCT) is a safe, effective, and sensitive imaging modality for detecting early-stage lung cancer and reduces mortality.
- The evolution of the Lung CT Screening Reporting and Data System has refined the clinician's ability to risk-stratify pulmonary nodules found on LDCT.
- Guidelines for lung cancer screening were based on enrollment criteria of clinical trials and have since been modified to capture more at-risk patients.
- Lung cancer screening is cost-effective but does potentiate cancer-related racial and socioeconomic disparity and exacerbate health inequity.

INTRODUCTION

Lung cancer is the leading cause of cancer-related deaths in the United States. In 2022, there were an estimated 236,740 new cases and 130,180 deaths. Five-year survival is estimated at 22.9%; however, when diagnosed early and appropriately treated, survival approaches 80%.[1,2] Approximately 80% to 90% of lung cancer deaths are associated with tobacco consumption, and the Centers for Disease Control and Prevention estimates that cigarette smokers have a 15- to 30-fold increased risk of developing primary lung cancer than never-smokers.[3] Islami and colleagues[4] calculated the cost of lost earnings for lung cancer to be approximately $21.3 billion for 2015; this is equal to the lost earnings of colorectal, breast, and pancreatic cancer combined. These sobering survival statistics and the substantial economic impact propelled the urgency for lung cancer screening (LCS) to the forefront of preventative care.

The impetus for LCS began in the 1950s with chest radiography (CXR) and sputum cytology. Over the next 2 decades, observational studies, including the American Cancer Society–Veterans Administration, South London Lung Cancer Study, and the Philadelphia Pulmonary Neoplasm Project, all reached the same conclusion: the survival of detected lung cancer in men was dismal, ranging between 8% and 18%.[5–8] Studies from Johns Hopkins, Mayo Clinic, and Memorial Sloan Kettering in the 1970s and the Prostate, Lung, Colorectal, and Ovarian trial in 1990 randomized CXR and sputum every 4 months compared with annual CXR. Unsurprisingly, as the method of detection had not changed, there was no difference in cancer mortality.[9–11] By 1990, computed tomographic (CT) scans emerged as a promising modality for lung cancer detection. Several studies, including the Anti-Lung Cancer Association Project in Japan and the Early Lung Cancer Action Project (ELCAP) in the United States, found

[a] Division of Thoracic Surgery, Department of Surgery, University of Cincinnati School of Medicine, 231 Albert Sabin Way Suite 2472, Cincinnati, OH 45267, USA; [b] Division of Thoracic Surgery, Department of Surgery, Duke University School of Medicine, Box 3531 DUMC, Durham, NC 27710, USA; [c] Division of Cardiothoracic Imaging, Department of Radiology, Duke University School of Medicine, Box 3808 DUMC, Durham, NC 27710, USA
* Corresponding author.
E-mail address: Hai.salfity@uc.edu

Thorac Surg Clin 33 (2023) 309–321
https://doi.org/10.1016/j.thorsurg.2023.04.001
1547-4127/23/Published by Elsevier Inc.

that most of the cancer diagnosed by CT scans were stage IA.[12,13] The International Early Lung Cancer Action Project (I-ELCAP), an expansion of ELCAP, estimated the 10-year survival of stage I lung cancer to be 88%.[14] This staggering result and new technology provided the necessary momentum for modern-day cancer screening trials (**Table 1**).

LOW-DOSE CHEST COMPUTED TOMOGRAPHY

Several prospective randomized trials using low-dose computed tomographic (LDCT) scans began in the early 2000s. These included the Lung Screening Study, Depiscan, UK Lung Cancer Screening Trial, Detection And screening of early lung cancer with Novel imaging Technology (DANTE), ITALUNG, The Danish Lung Cancer Screening Trial (DLCST), and LUSI.[15–22] The studies compared LDCT with either CXR or usual care, varied in inclusion criteria (eg, age, smoking histories, lung cancer risks), and had average follow-up of 4 to 5 years. The findings were similar: (1) using LDCT to detect lung cancer was feasible, but (2) lung cancer found at an earlier stage had little impact on mortality (**Table 2**).

Although the studied population ranged from several hundred to 4099 patients, it was clear that these trials were inadequately powered to detect the mortality benefit associated with LCS. Meanwhile, the National Lung Screening Trial (NLST), conducted in the United States, enrolled 53,454 patients between the ages of 55 and 74 years, had a smoking history of at least 30 pack-years (PY; [pack(s) per day × number of years]), and were currently smoking or quit within 15 years.[23–25] Nearly 50% of cancers detected by LDCT in NLST were stage I. More importantly,

lung cancer–related mortality was reduced by 20%, and overall mortality was reduced by 6.7%. Similarly, the Nederlands–Leuvens Longkanker Screenings Onderzoek (NELSON) Trial, conducted in the Netherlands and Belgium, enrolled 15,792 patients and reported a 26% reduction in lung cancer mortality after 10 years of screening.[23–25] The findings of NLST and NELSON justified the benefit of using LDCT as an effective screening test for lung cancer. Shortly thereafter, professional societies, including the National Comprehensive Cancer Network (NCCN), the American College of Chest Physicians (ACCP), and the American Cancer Society, began publishing guidelines for wide implementation of LCS. In 2013, the United States Preventive Services Task Force (USPSTF) released a grade B recommendation for yearly LCS with LDCT in individuals at high risk for lung cancer.[26]

ESTABLISHMENT AND EVOLUTION OF LUNG COMPUTED TOMOGRAPHIC SCREENING REPORTING AND DATA SYSTEM

Following publication of the NLST[23] and the 2013 USPSTF recommendations,[26] there was growing interest in effective LCS implementation, particularly regarding safe LDCT acquisition, standardized interpretation, and downstream management.[27] In response, the American College of Radiology (ACR) developed the Lung CT Screening Reporting and Data System (Lung-RADS), which was modeled after the Breast Imaging Reporting and Data System. Lung-RADS version 1.0 was released in 2014; version 1.1 was issued in 2019, and the updated Lung-RADS 2022 was released in November 2022.[28]

Lung-RADS standardized reporting of LDCTs, defining categories for negative and positive

---

Table 1
Lung cancer screening trials using plain chest radiography and sputum cytology

	Study Period	No. of Participants	Age (y)	Smoking History (ppd)	Duration (y)	Mortality
Mayo Lung Project	1971–1976	9211	≥45	≥1	6	NS
Johns Hopkins Lung Project	1973–1978	10,387	≥45	≥1	5	NS
Memorial Sloan Kettering Lung Study	1974–1978	10,040	≥45	≥1	5	NS
Prostate, Lung, Colorectal, and Ovary	1993–2001	154,901	55–74	—	3	NS

All studies compared annual chest X ray ± sputum cytology with annual chest X ray alone.
Abbreviations: NS, not significant; ppd, pack(s) per day.

Table 2
Lung cancer screening trials using low-dose computed tomography

	Country	Study Period	No. of Participants	Age (y)	Smoking History	Duration	Cancer Mortality	Overall Mortality
Lung Screening Study (LSS)	USA	2000	3318	55–74	≥30 PY Current or former smoker within 10 y	N/A	NS	NS
Depiscan	France	2002–2004	765	50–75	≥15 cigs/d × ≥20 y; current or former smoker within 15 y	2 y	—	—
UK Lung Cancer Screening Trial	United Kingdom	2011	4055	50–75	a	N/A	—	—
DANTE	Italy	2001–2006	2532	60–74	≥20 PY	4 y	NS	
ITALUNG	Italy	2003–2007	3206	55–69	≥20 PY	3 y	NS	
National Lung Screening Trial (NLST)	USA	2002–2004	53,454	55–74	≥30 PY Current or former smoker within 15 y	2 y	20% reduction	6.7% reduction
NELSON	Netherlands Belgium	2000–2004	15,792	50–75	≥15 cigs/d × 25 y ≥10 cigs/d × ≥30 y	5.5 y	26% reduction	NS
Danish Lung Cancer Screening Trial (DLCST)	Denmark	2004–2006	4104	50–70	≥20 PY Current or former smoker	4 y	NS	—
Multicentric Italian Lung Detection (MILD)	Italy	2005–2011	4099	≥49	≥20 PY Current or former smoker within 10 y	6 y	39% reduction	20% reduction
LUSI	Germany	2007–2011	4052	50–69	≥15 cigs/d × 25 y; ≥10 cigs/d × ≥ 30 y; current or former smoker within 10 y	4 y	Reduction in women (HR, 0.31); NS in men	—

All studies were compared with standard of care as defined by the country or plain chest radiography.
Abbreviations: —, not reported; cigs, cigarettes; N/A, not applicable; NS, nonsignificant.
a Participants must have a 5-y lung cancer risk ≥5% according to the Liverpool Lung Project Risk model.

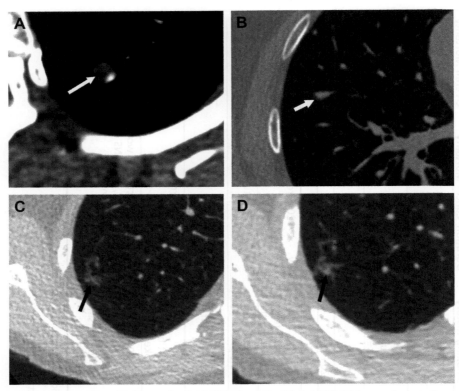

Fig. 1. Lung-RADS category 1 and 2 ("negative") LDCT LCS results. (A) Axial LDCT demonstrates a 9-mm nodule in the left upper lobe with macroscopic fat (*arrow*) compatible with a benign pulmonary hamartoma (category 1). (B) 9-mm perifissural nodule along the right major fissure with characteristic smooth margins and a triangular shape (*arrow*) (category 2). (C) Baseline LDCT with a 1.8 x 0.8 cm predominantly pure GGN (*arrow*) (category 2 by Lung-RADS 1.1). (D) On repeat annual CT, the purely GGN in **Fig. 1**C developed a small solid nodular component, upgrading it to a category 4A (*arrow*). The interval change suggests a low-grade adenocarcinoma-spectrum neoplasm and is confirmed by tissue diagnosis.

results and linking these categories with follow-up recommendations. Central to Lung-RADS was the need to effectively define the threshold for positive screens, balancing test sensitivity with the risk of false-positive examination. The latter was of particular concern, given that 96.4% of positive LDCT screenings in the NLST were false positives.[23] The NLST defined a positive LDCT screening examination as a solid nodule ≥4 mm. Lung-RADS defines it as ≥6 mm.[28] This increase in size threshold was supported by data from the I-ELCAP and retrospective reevaluation of the NLST demonstrating that an increased threshold would reduce false positives with relatively small sensitivity reductions.[27,29,30] Pinsky and colleagues[30] demonstrated that applying Lung-RADS 1.0 to the LDCT arm of the NLST reduced false positive rates from 26.6% to 12.8% at baseline and 21.8% to 5.3% on repeat LCS with corresponding small decreases in test sensitivity.

In addition to nodule size, Lung-RADS uses imaging features for nodule characterization.

Category 1 and 2 findings are "negative," including LDCTs without nodules, nodules with benign calcification patterns or intralesional fat, solid nodules ≤6 mm at baseline LDCT, ground-glass nodules (GGN) less than 30 mm, juxtapleural nodules less than 10 mm (with typical characteristics of intrapulmonary lymph nodes), and airway-associated abnormalities typical of secretions/mucous plugs (**Fig. 1**). Characterization of the latter 3 items has evolved over the iterations of Lung-RADS. For instance, allowable size thresholds for perifissural nodules and GGNs increased between Lung-RADS 1.0 and Lung-RADS 1.1.[31] Lung-RADS 2022 further extended the definition of perifissural nodules to include all less than 10-mm juxtapleural nodules (ie, perifissural, costal pleural, perimediastinal/peridiaphragmatic) with smooth margins and triangular, lentiform, or ovoid shape, as likely benign intrapulmonary lymph nodes.[32,33] Also, whereas prior versions of Lung-RADS considered all endobronchial

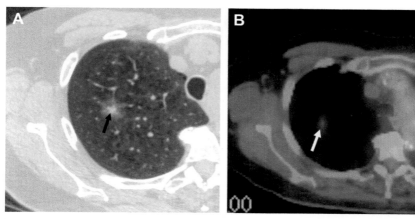

Fig. 2. Positive LCS with a part-solid nodule. (*A*) Baseline LCS with a part-solid nodule measuring 2.0 × 1.5 cm and a central solid component (*arrow*) measuring 0.9 cm (category 4B). (*B*) PET/CT shows mild fluorodeoxyglucose (FDG) -avidity in the right upper lobe nodule (*arrow*) with a maximum standardized uptake value of 1.2. Surgical wedge resection confirmed invasive acinar adenocarcinoma.

nodules as "positive" screens, Lung-RADS 2022 characterizes subsegmental and certain proximal airway abnormalities with internal air, lack of significant soft tissue, and lack of obstruction as negative findings, as transient secretions and likely benign.[34] Importantly, although Lung-RADS category 2 results are considered "negative," this should not be taken to mean that the individual does not have cancer; rather, the result indicates a low likelihood of a clinically active neoplasm and continued annual LCS should be pursued (**Fig. 1**C, D).

Lung-RADS 3, 4A, 4B, and 4X classifications are positive results (**Figs. 2** and **3**) necessitating follow-up via 6-month (category 3) or 3-month LDCT (category 4A). For 4B and 4X lesions, additional testing includes PET/CT, tissue sampling, or follow-up diagnostic chest CT with or without contrast (see **Fig. 3**). Recognizing that some neoplasms, particularly adenocarcinomas, may

have cystic features, the concept of atypical pulmonary cysts was formally introduced into Lung-RADS 2022.[35,36] Such cysts may be classified as Lung-RADS 3/4A/4B, depending on features like a thickened wall, multilocularity, or nodular components (**Fig. 4**). Another salient update to Lung-RADS 2022 included the management of infectious/inflammatory nodules, which are approximately 10% of false positive LDCTs[37,38] (**Fig. 5**). Lung-RADS 1.1[39] characterized new, large opacities suspected to be inflammatory or infectious as category 4B lesions with the recommendation for a 1-month follow-up CT to assess for resolution. However, Lung-RADS 2022 permits these lesions to be classified as category 0 or 2, thereby circumventing a "positive" LCS result. Future work is needed to determine how this change affects LCS outcomes, particularly regarding false positive and false negative rates.

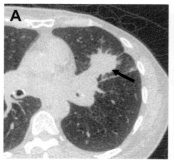
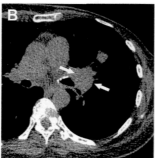
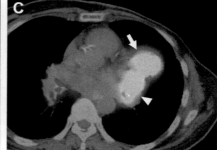

Fig. 3. Lung-RADS category 4X lesion. (*A*) Baseline axial LDCT shows a spiculated mass in the left upper lobe (*black arrow*). (*B*) Axial images demonstrate ipsilateral left hilar adenopathy (*white arrows*) suspicious for nodal metastasis (category 4X). (*C*) PET/CT shows FDG-avidity in the dominant mass (*white arrow*) and in the left hilar lymphadenopathy (*arrowhead*). Tissue biopsy confirmed adenocarcinoma.

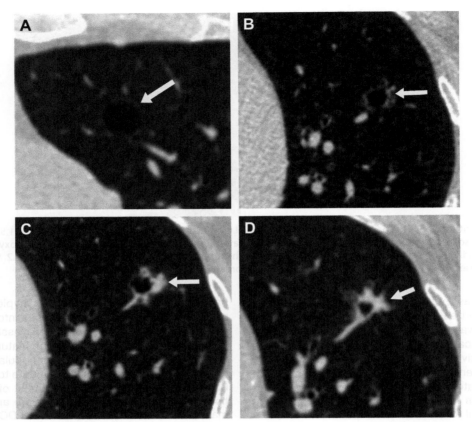

Fig. 4. Cystic lesions. (*A*) Thin-walled cyst with wall thickness less than 2 mm and smooth borders (*arrow*). These are benign and not managed by Lung-RADS. (*B*) Baseline CT shows an irregular cyst with total diameter measuring 1.2 cm and an irregular asymmetric thickened wall (*arrow*) measuring up to 4 mm (atypical pulmonary cyst, category 4A). (*C*) Follow-up CT at 6 months revealed a growing soft tissue component (*arrow*). (*D*) CT at 9 months revealed continued increase in the solid component (*arrow*).

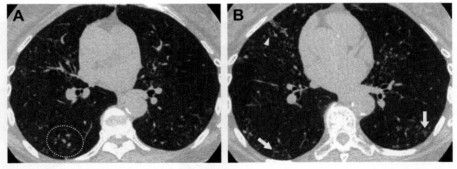

Fig. 5. Infectious nodules. (*A*) Multiple bilateral nodules at baseline LCS with the largest cluster in the right lower lobe measuring up to 6 mm (*circle*). (*B*) Images from the same CT demonstrate additional smaller centrilobular nodules in a tree-in-bud configuration (*arrows*) with mild bronchiectasis in the right middle lobe (*arrowhead*). This constellation of findings suggests a chronic nontuberculous mycobacterial infection. Lung-RADS 1.1 classified the 6-mm nodule as a "positive" with category 4A. Lung-RADS 2022 classified this as category 0 or 2.

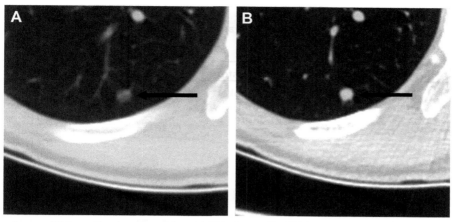

Fig. 6. Importance of thin-section imaging. (*A*) Axial CT in 5-mm slice thickness demonstrates a 3-mm nodule with apparent ground-glass consistency (*arrow*). (*B*) Thin-section image with axial thickness of 1.25 mm demonstrates that the nodule is solid (*arrow*). Thin-section imaging is a requisite for accurate characterization of nodule consistency and provides the necessary spatial resolution for accurate nodule measurement.

FUNDAMENTAL IMAGING CONSIDERATIONS

LDCT acquisition must ensure sufficient imaging quality for assessment of small pulmonary nodules while also minimizing radiation.[40] The ACR–Society of Thoracic Radiology Practice Parameter for the Performance and Reporting of Lung Cancer Screening Thoracic Computed Tomography and the American Association of Physicists in Medicine have published technical guidelines for LDCT acquisition.[41,42]

Acquisition and Low-Dose Parameters

LDCT is performed with a multidetector ($\geq$16 detector rows) helical technique in full inspiration with a single breath-hold. Axial images are acquired from the lung apices through the costophrenic sulci and viewed at $\leq$2.5-mm slice thickness[41,42] (**Fig. 6**). Thin-section ($\leq$1 mm) reconstructions may increase sensitivity of nodule detection and characterization.[42–44]

The low-dose radiation parameters in adherence with "as low as reasonably achievable" (ALARA) principles are applied to screening CT. A dose index volume ($CTDI_{vol}$) should be $\leq$3 mGy, must be used with scanner output adjustment, and must be adjusted for patient's size.[41,42] The estimated effective dose for an LDCT is 1.0 mSv or less,[42] and the cumulative increased risk of cancer after 20 annual LDCTs would be 0.22% in women and 0.12% in men.[40] These risks are substantially smaller than the estimated lifetime risk of lung cancer development: 6.7% and 5.9% among smoking and nonsmoking individuals, respectively.[1]

UNITED STATES PREVENTIVE SERVICES TASK FORCE RECOMMENDATIONS AND INSURANCE COVERAGE

The eligibility criteria from the 2013 USPSTF guidelines for LCS using LDCT were as follows: asymptomatic individuals between 55 and 80 years of age with a greater than 30 PY smoking history who are currently smoking or have quit smoking within the past 15 years.[26] Categorized as a grade B preventive service, LDCT is, therefore, covered by all private insurers without cost-sharing as dictated by the US Affordable Care Act.[45,46] In 2015, the Centers for Medicare and Medicaid Services (CMS) released a decision memo to provide LDCT LCS to Medicare beneficiaries as a preventive health benefit.[47] CMS selection criteria, however, included an upper age limit of 77 years, which was more congruent with recommendations by the ACCP[48] and the NCCN[49] at that time (**Table 3**).

Since the implementation of screening programs, several barriers have arisen. Most notably, LCS utilization rate remains less than 20% nationwide.[50–54] In contrast, colorectal, breast, and cervical cancer screening adherence rates range consistently around 60% in eligible populations.[55] Moreover, the 2013 LCS eligibility criteria, which were modeled after the NLST, only captured 27% of the actual at-risk patient population and 16% of eligible black patients.[50] The biggest limitations are the PYs and the smoking cessation of 15 years or less.[56] In 2021, the USPSTF revised the LCS eligibility criteria with salient changes as follows: (1) the minimum age for screening enrollment was lowered to 50 years; and (2) the

Table 3
Previous and current recommendations for lung cancer screening in the United States

	Previous Recommendations		New Recommendations	
	Age Range (y)	Smoking History	Age Range (y)	Smoking History
USPSTF	55–80	Current smoker Quit within 15 y 30 PY or greater	50–80	Current smoker Quit within 15 y 20 PY or greater
CMS	55–77		50–80	Current smoker Quit within 15 y 20 PY or greater
NCCN	55–77		≥50	20 PY or greater
ACCP	55–77		55–77	Current smoker Quit within 15 y 30 PY or greater
AATS	55–79	30 PY or greater	55–79	30 PY or greater

Abbreviation: AATS, American Association for Thoracic Surgery .

minimum PY was decreased to 20.[47] In 2022, CMS expanded coverage in accordance with the 2021 USPSTF guidelines[48] (see **Table 3**).

Within the original 2015 decision memo, CMS required shared decision making (SDM) between provider and patient, counseling on LCS risks and benefits, and smoking-cessation discussions.[57,58] The provider must be a physician or a midlevel advanced practitioner (APP).[57] Because only 75% of Americans have primary care physicians (PCP) and less so for patients who are in the third to sixth decade of life, LCS is not readily available to everyone at risk.[59] The memo also required specific criteria for imaging facilities and interpreting radiologists and mandatory reporting to a national LCS registry. To date, the ACR Lung Cancer Screening Registry serves as the repository for these data but with limited access for outcome analyses.[60] These mandates were scrutinized for creating unnecessary administrative burden without improving quality of care, all the while limiting access to screening.[47] Recent provisions have abolished the national registry reporting requirements and allowed SDM to be performed by clinical nursing staff.[48] It remains to be seen whether this will increase LCS utilization rates.

It is important to mention that these coverage determinations only applied to those with insurance. For the uninsured, who are disproportionately affected by lung cancer, the costs of LDCT and downstream care are unlikely to be affordable.[61–63] The lack of third-party payor support for patients less than 65 years of age has been a large deterrent to enrollment in LCS.[56,61] The 2022 National Health Statistics Reports found that greater than 15% of adults less than 65 years

are uninsured.[64] These issues are prominent in colorectal and breast cancer screening, and LCS will likely have the same disparate trajectory. There are no provisions, past or current, to address this problem.

CONTROVERSIES OF LUNG CANCER SCREENING

Criticisms of LCS are many and have evolved as the program continues to mature. Historically, the critique centers on inadequate modality (ie, CXR) for cancer detection, which translates to minimal impact on cancer mortality. As diagnostic imaging becomes increasingly sensitive, the pendulum has oscillated to overdiagnosis, high false positive rates, lifetime radiation dose, and incidental findings resulting in unnecessary procedures and risks. Additional trepidations include concerns over cost-effectiveness, health disparities, and the anxiety associated with the diagnosis of an unspecified or indeterminate pulmonary nodule.[61]

Psychological Impact

Costs associated with false positive results and overdiagnosis (estimated to be 18% in screen-detected cancers in NLST)[65] extend beyond the procedure-related implications.[66] The results, whether positive or falsely positive, induce significant stress and anxiety. In the NELSON trial, cancer-specific distress was noted to be higher in patients with false positive findings despite no changes noted on the overall health-related quality-of-life measurements.[67,68] In the wake of the current mental health epidemic, it is important to address these issues and integrate psychosocial support and counseling to those enrolled in LCS programs.

Cost-Effectiveness

Upon the issuance of the USPSTF guidelines, a series of studies began to explore the cost-effectiveness of LCS.[69–72] Analysis of NLST by Black and colleagues[69] noted that LDCT is cost-effective compared with no cancer screening, assuming the generated economic model stays relatively constant. This is corroborated by a systematic review from Puggina and colleagues[70] whereby LCS generated an incremental cost-effectiveness ratio (ICERs) of less than $100,000 per quality-adjusted life year (QALY) gained (cost-effectiveness benchmark). Furthermore, higher-risk populations (eg, Medicare beneficiaries, older patients) with higher PYs have lower ICERs per QALY gained. It is, therefore, more cost-effective to screen current smokers ($116,000 per QALY gained) than former smokers ($2,322,700 per QALY gained).[70,71] Similarly, LDCT screening of never-smokers in the United States is not cost-effective, generating ICERs of $3 million per QALY gained for men and $2 million per QALY gained for women.[72]

In addition, the financial expenditures relating to incidental findings and associated procedures need to be taken into consideration. Multiple studies noted that treatment of pure GGNs or incidentally discovered nodules on coronary CT angiography are not cost-effective with ICERs of $129,800 per QALY gained for smokers alone.[73,74] Meanwhile, the relative reduction in mortality was only 4.6%.[74] Similarly, although Gilbert and colleagues[75] reported that an incidental pulmonary nodule clinic coupled with an APP can increase revenue streams for a single hospital system, there were no evidence of cost-effectiveness. These studies collectively suggest that a nonstructured LCS program without adherence to screening criteria exudes little economic benefit. This ultimately gives weight to some of the recommendations as set forth by the USPSTF.

Lung Cancer Screening Acceptance

The harshest critic of LCS has been the American Academy of Family Physicians (AAFP). Shortly after the 2013 USPSTF recommendations, the AAFP issued an official statement claiming that current evidence was not sufficient to endorse or oppose the use of LDCT for LCS.[76] That stance played a major role in the promotion of LCS in the United States. A survey performed in 2016 noted that only 36% of PCPs in South Carolina were aware of the frequency for LCS, whereas greater than

60% were not familiar with LDCT insurance coverage. Physicians were also uninformed about recommendations from other professional societies and had no formal training on the structure of LCS.[77] As a result, LCS was still not offered as a preventative service in more than 1500 PCP offices by 2018.[78] Because studies have shown that the participation of PCP is associated with improved population health outcomes, the AAFP stance was detrimental to the initial development of LCS.

In 2021, the AAFP, now citing sufficient evidence despite no new trials, officially endorsed LDCT for LCS.[79] The current endorsement, although welcomed, will require educational training for PCPs and will ultimately take several years to see the full effects on the acceptance of LCS.

SUMMARY

LCS has evolved since its inception 70 years ago. Technological advancements have allowed for early detection with relatively low risk. The development of the Lung-RADS classification has further refined the diagnostic and surveillance criteria. So far, the benefits of LCS outweigh the risks. The next steps will be to systematically implement an effective and efficient program: one that will benefit patients, address the ever-expanding health care expenditure, and improve health equity. It is no ordinary feat, but we are up for the challenge.

CLINICS CARE POINTS

- On low-dose computed tomography obtained for the purpose of lung cancer screening, the recommendations must include a Lung CT Screening Reporting and Data System grading.

- On reviewing low-dose computed tomography, a growing nodule is defined by greater than 1.5 mm of growth in the mean diameter within a 12-month interval and should have short-term follow-up imaging.

- On low-dose computed tomography with Lung CT Screening Reporting and Data System 3 findings, a follow-up scan should be obtained within 6 months. If findings are stable or decreased, the study should be reclassified as Lung CT Screening Reporting and Data System 2 and return to annual screening from the date of the most recent examination.

- On low-dose computed tomography with Lung CT Screening Reporting and Data System 4A findings, a follow-up scan should be obtained within 3 months. If findings are stable or decreased, the study should be reclassified as Lung CT Screening Reporting and Data System 3 with appropriate follow-up (6 months from date of most current examination). If imaging remains stable, then the study would be down-graded to Lung CT Screening Reporting and Data System 2 with accordant follow-up.

- When encountered by individuals who are symptomatic, do not suggest lung cancer screening. These patients require diagnostic computed tomographic scans.

- Plain chest radiography is an inappropriate lung cancer screening tool and should not be offered to patients as an alternative to low-dose computed tomography.

- When encountering patients who do not meet lung cancer screening criteria as set out by the United States Preventive Services Task Force or Centers for Medicare and Medicaid Services, patients need to be counseled on the out-of-pocket costs of the scan. This cost is institution dependent.

- During the discussion with patients regarding the risks and benefits of low-dose computed tomography, providers/nurse navigators should document the shared decision-making process with the patient whereby patient and providers/nurse navigators arrived at the decision to pursue low-dose computed tomography together.

- During the discussion with patients regarding the risks and benefits of low-dose computed tomography, providers/nurse navigators should discuss smoking cessation counseling.

- When discussing low-dose computed tomography and lung cancer screening with patients, providers should accurately document the pack-year smoking histories and years since smoking cessation has occurred.

- When discussing the advantages and disadvantages of lung cancer screening, it is not cost-effective to screen never-smokers.

DISCLOSURE

The authors have nothing to disclose.

REFERENCES

1. Siegel RL, Miller KD, Fuchs HE, et al. Cancer statistics, 2022. CA Cancer J Clin 2022;72:7–33.

2. Cancer and Stat Facts: Lung and Bronchus Cancer. National Cancer Institute, 2022. Available at: https://seer.cancer.gov/statfacts/html/lungb.html. Accessed January 19, 2023.

3. Lung Cancer: what are the risk factors for lung cancer. Division of Cancer Prevention and Control, Centers for Disease Control and Prevention, 2022. Available at: https://www.cdc.gov/cancer/lung/basic_info/risk_factors.htm#:~:text=Cigarette%20smoking%20is%20the%20number,the%20risk%20for%20lung%20cancer. Accessed January 19, 2023.

4. Islami F, Miller KD, Siegel RL, et al. National and state estimates of lost earnings from cancer deaths in the United States. JAMA Oncol 2019;5(9):e191460.

5. Yabroff KR, Mariotto A, Tangka F, et al. Annual Report to the Nation on the Status of Cancer, Part 2: Patient Economic Burden Associated With Cancer Care. Journal of the National Cancer Institute 2021;113(12):1670–82.

6. Nash FA, Morgan JM, Tomkins JG. South London Lung Cancer Study. Br Med J 1968;2:715–21.

7. Lilienfeld A, Archer PG, Burnett CH, et al. An evaluation of radiologic and cytologic screening for the early detection of lung cancer: a cooperative pilot study of the American Cancer Society and Veterans Administration. Cancer Res 1966;26:2083–121.

8. Weiss W, Boucot KR, Cooper DA. The Philadelphia pulmonary neoplasm research project. Survival factors in bronchogenic carcinoma. JAMA 1971;216:2119–23.

9. Berlin NI, Buncher CR, Fontana RS, et al. The National Cancer Institute Cooperative Early Lung Cancer Detection Program. Results of the initial screen (prevalence). Early lung cancer detection: Introduction. Am Rev Respir Dis 1984;130:545–9.

10. Marcus PM, Bergstralh EJ, Fagerstrom RM, et al. Lung cancer mortality in the Mayo Lung Project: impact of extended follow-up. J Natl Cancer Inst 2000;92:1308–16.

11. Oken MM, Hocking WG, Kvale PA, et al. Screening by chest radiograph and lung cancer mortality: the Prostate, Lung, Colorectal, and Ovarian (PLCO) randomized trial. JAMA 2011;306:1865–73.

12. Sobue T, Moriyama N, Kaneko M, et al. Screening for lung cancer with low-dose helical computed tomography: anti-lung cancer association project. J Clin Oncol 2002;20:911–20.

13. Henschke CI, McCauley DI, Yankelevitz DF, et al. Early Lung Cancer Action Project: overall design and findings from baseline screening. Lancet 1999;354:99–105.

14. Henschke CI, Yankelevitz DF, Libby DM, et al, International Early Lung Cancer Action Program I. Survival of patients with stage I lung cancer detected on CT screening. N Engl J Med 2006;355:1763–71.

15. Blanchon T, Brechot JM, Grenier PA, et al. Baseline results of the Depiscan study: a French randomized pilot trial of lung cancer screening comparing low dose CT scan (LDCT) and chest X-ray (CXR). Lung Cancer 2007;58:50–8.

16. Field JK, Duffy SW, Baldwin DR, et al. UK Lung Cancer RCT Pilot Screening Trial: baseline findings from the screening arm provide evidence for the potential implementation of lung cancer screening. Thorax 2016;71:161–70.

17. Gohagan JK, Marcus PM, Fagerstrom RM, et al. Final results of the Lung Screening Study, a randomized feasibility study of spiral CT versus chest X-ray screening for lung cancer. Lung Cancer 2005;47:9–15.

18. Infante M, Cavuto S, Lutman FR, et al. Long-Term Follow-up Results of the DANTE Trial, a Randomized Study of Lung Cancer Screening with Spiral Computed Tomography. Am J Respir Crit Care Med 2015;191:1166–75.

19. Paci E, Puliti D, Lopes Pegna A, et al. Mortality, survival and incidence rates in the ITALUNG randomised lung cancer screening trial. Thorax 2017;72: 825–31.

20. Saghir Z, Dirksen A, Ashraf H, et al. CT screening for lung cancer brings forward early disease. The randomised Danish Lung Cancer Screening Trial: status after five annual screening rounds with low-dose CT. Thorax 2012;67:296–301.

21. Wille MM, Dirksen A, Ashraf H, et al. Results of the Randomized Danish Lung Cancer Screening Trial with Focus on High-Risk Profiling. Am J Respir Crit Care Med 2016;193:542–51.

22. Becker N, Motsch E, Trotter A, et al. Lung cancer mortality reduction by LDCT screening-Results from the randomized German LUSI trial. Int J Cancer 2020;146:1503–13.

23. Aberle DR, Adams AM, Berg CD, et al. National Lung Screening Trial Research Team, Reduced lung-cancer mortality with low-dose computed tomographic screening. N Engl J Med 2011;365: 395–409.

24. van Iersel CA, de Koning HJ, Draisma G, et al. Risk-based selection from the general population in a screening trial: selection criteria, recruitment and power for the Dutch-Belgian randomised lung cancer multi-slice CT screening trial (NELSON). Int J Cancer 2007;120:868–74.

25. de Koning HJ, van der Aalst CM, de Jong PA, et al. Reduced Lung-Cancer Mortality with Volume CT Screening in a Randomized Trial. N Engl J Med 2020;382:503–13.

26. US Preventive Services Task Force, Moyer VA. Screening for Lung Cancer: US Preventive Services Task Force Recommendation Statement. Ann Intern Med 2014;160:330–8.

27. Gierada DS, Pinsky P, Nath H, et al. Projected outcomes using different nodule sizes to define a positive CT lung cancer screening examination. J Natl Cancer Inst 2014;106:dju284.

28. Lung-Screening Reporting and Data System (LungRADS) version 2022. Available at: https://www.acr.org/Clinical-Resources/Reporting-and-Data-Systems/Lung-Rads. Accessed January 19, 2023.

29. Henschke C, Yip R. Yankelevitz D.F., et al., Definition of a positive test result in computed tomography screening for lung cancer: a cohort study. Ann Intern Med 2013;158(4):246–52.

30. Pinsky PF, Gierada DS, Black W, et al. Performance of Lung-RADS in the National Lung Screening Trial: a retrospective assessment. Ann Intern Med 2015; 162(7):485–91.

31. Kastner J, Hossain R, Jeudy J, et al. Lung-RADS Version 1.0 versus Lung-RADS Version 1.1: Comparison of Categories Using Nodules from the National Lung Screening Trial. Radiology 2021;300(1): 199–206.

32. Schreuder A, van Ginneken B, Scholten ET, et al. Classification of CT Pulmonary Opacities as Perifissural Nodules: Reader Variability. Radiology 2018; 288(3):867–75.

33. Mets OM, Chung K, Scholten ET, et al. Incidental perifissural nodules on routine chest computed tomography: lung cancer or not? Eur Radiol 2018; 28(3):1095–101.

34. Kim HJ, Kim DK, Kim YW, et al. Outcome of incidentally detected airway nodules. Eur Respir J 2016; 47(5):1510–7.

35. Mendoza DP, Heeger A, Mino-Kenudson M, et al. Clinicopathologic and Longitudinal Imaging Features of Lung Cancer Associated With Cystic Airspaces: A Systematic Review and Meta-Analysis. AJR 2021;216(2):318–29.

36. Farooqi A.O., Cham M., Zhang L., et al., International Early Lung Cancer Action Program Investigators, Lung cancer associated with cystic airspaces, Am J Roentgenol, 199 (4), 2012, 781– 786.

37. Mendoza DP, Chintanapakdee W, Zhang EW, et al. Management and outcomes of suspected infectious and inflammatory lung abnormalities identified on lung cancer screening CT. AJR 2021;217:5.

38. ZhaoY.R., Heuvelmans M.A., Dorrius M.D., et al., Features of resolving and nonresolving indeterminate pulmonary nodules at follow-up CT: the NELSON study, Radiology, 270 (3), 2014, 872–879.

39. Lung-RADS Version 1.1. American College of Radiology. Available at: https://www.acr.org/-/media/ACR/Files/RADS/Lung-RADS/LungRADSAssessmentCategoriesv1-1.pdf. 2019. Accessed January 19, 2023.

40. Gierada DS, Black WC, Chiles C, et al. Low-dose CT screening for lung cancer: evidence from 2 decades of study. Radiology: Imaging Cancer 2020;2(2): e190058.

41. ACR-STR Practice Parameter for the Performance and Reporting of Lung Cancer Screening Thoracic Computed Tomography. Available at https://www.acr.org/-/media/ACR/Files/Practice-Parameters/CT-LungCaScr.pdf?la=en. Accessed January 19, 2023.

42. American Association of Physicists in Medicine. Lung Cancer Screening Protocols Version 4.0. Available at: https://www.aapm.org/pubs/CTProtocols/documents/LungCancerScreeningCT.pdf. Published 2019. Accessed January 19, 2023.

43. Jankowski A, Martinelli T, Timsit JF, et al. Pulmonary nodule detection on MDCT images: evaluation of diagnostic performance using thin axial images, maximum intensity projections, and computer-assisted detection. Eur Radiol 2007;17(12):3148–56.

44. Kawel N, Seifert B, Luetolf M, et al. Effect of slab thickness on the CT detection of pulmonary nodules: use of sliding thin-slab maximum intensity projection and volume rendering. Am J Roentgenol 2009;192(5):1324–9.

45. Coverage of Certain Preventive Services Under the Affordable Care Act. 2015. Available at: https://www.federalregister.gov/documents/2015/07/14/2015-17076/coverage-of-certain-preventive-services-under-the-affordable-care-act. Accessed January 19, 2023.

46. Zhao J, Mao Z, Fedewa SA, et al. The Affordable Care Act and access to care across the cancer control continuum: A review at 10 years. CA A Cancer J Clin 2020;70(3):165–81.

47. US Preventive Services Task Force, Krist AH, Davidson KW, et al. Screening for Lung Cancer: US Preventive Services Task Force Recommendation Statement. JAMA 2021;325(10):962.

48. Decision memo for screening for lung cancer with low dose computed tomography (LDCT) (CAG-00439R). Available at: https://www.cms.gov/medicare-coverage-database/view/ncacal-decision-memo.aspx?proposed=N&ncaid=304. Accessed January 19, 2023.

49. Wood DE, Kazerooni EA, Baum SL, et al. Lung Cancer Screening, Version 3.2018, NCCN Clinical Practice Guidelines in Oncology. J Natl Compr Canc Netw 2018;16:412–41.

50. Zgodic A, Zahnd WE, Miller DP Jr, et al. Predictors of Lung Cancer Screening Utilization in a Population-Based Survey. JACR 2020;17(12):1591–601.

51. Zahnd WE, Eberth JM. Lung Cancer Screening Utilization: A behavioral risk factor surveillance system analysis. Am J Prev Med 2019;57(2):250–5.

52. Zgodic A, Zahnd WE, Advani S, et al. Low-dose CT lung cancer screening uptake: a rural-urban comparison. J Rural Health 2022;38(1):40–53.

53. Jemal A, Fedewa SA. Lung Cancer Screening With Low-Dose Computed Tomography in the United States-2010 to 2015. JAMA Oncol 2017;3:1278–81.

54. Tailor TD, Tong BC, Gao J, et al. Utilization of Lung Cancer Screening in the Medicare Fee-for-Service Population. Chest 2020;158(5):2200–10.

55. Closing Gaps in Cancer Screening: Connecting people, communities, and systems to improve equity and access. February 2022. Available at: https://prescancerpanel.cancer.gov/report/cancerscreening/. Accessed January 19, 2023.

56. Pu CY, Lusk CM, Neslund-Dudas C, et al. Comparison Between the 2021 USPSTF Lung Cancer Screening Criteria and other lung cancer screening criteria for racial disparity in Eligibility. JAMA Oncol 2022;8(3):374–82.

57. Jensen T.S., Chin J., Ashby L., et al., Decision memo for screening for lung cancer with low dose computed tomography (LDCT) (CAG-00439N). Available at: https://www.cms.gov/medicare-coverage-database/details/nca-decision-memo.aspx?NCAId=274. Accessed January 19, 2023.

58. Mazzone PJ, Silvestri GA, Patel S, et al. Screening for Lung Cancer: CHEST Guideline and Expert Panel Report. Chest 2018;153:954–85.

59. Levine DM, Linder JA, Landon BE. Characteristics of Americans with primary care and changes over time, 2002-2015. JAMA Intern Med 2020;180(3):463–6.

60. ACR Website. Available at: https://www.acr.org/Practice-Management-Quality-Informatics/Registries/Lung-Cancer-Screening-Registry/FAQ. Accessed January 19, 2023.

61. Mulshine JL, D'Amico TD. Issues with implementing a high-quality lung cancer screening program. CA Cancer J Clin 2014;64:351–63.

62. Febbo J, Little B, Fischl-Lanzoni N, et al. Analysis of out-of-pocket cost of lung cancer screening for uninsured patients among ACR-accredited imaging centers. JACR 2020;17(9):1108–15.

63. Reese TJ, Schlechter CR, Potter LN, et al. Evaluation of Revised US Preventive Services Task Force Lung Cancer Screening Guideline Among Women and Racial/Ethnic Minority Populations. JAMA Netw Open 2021;4(1):e2033769.

64. Lee A., Ruhter J., Peters C., et al., National Uninsured Rate Reaches Al-time Low in Early 2022. (Brief No. HP-2022-23). U.S. Department of Health and Human Services. August 2022. Available at: https://aspe.hhs.gov/sites/default/files/documents/15c1f9899b3f203887deba90e3005f5a/Uninsured-Q1-2022-Data-Point-HP-2022-23-08.pdf. Accessed January 19, 2023.

65. Patz EF Jr, Pinsky P, Gatsonis C, et al. Overdiagnosis in low-dose computed tomography screening for lung cancer. JAMA Intern Med 2014;174(2):269–74. published correction appears in JAMA Intern Med. 2014 May;174(5):828.

66. Crosswell JM, Baker SG, Marcus PM, et al. Cumulative incidence of false-positive test results in lung

cancer screening. Annals of internal medicine 2010;
152:505–12.

67. Gareen IF, Duan F, Greco EM, et al. Impact of lung
cancer screening results on participant health-
related quality of life and state anxiety in the National
Lung Screening Trial. Cancer 2014;120:3401–9.

68. van den Bergh KA, Essink-Bot ML, Borsboom GJ,
et al. Short-term health-related quality of life consequences in a lung cancer CT screening trial
(NELSON). Br J Cancer 2010;102:27–34.

69. Black WC, Gareen IF, Soneji SS, et al. Cost-effectiveness of CT screening in the National Lung Screening
Trial. N Engl J Med 2014;371:1793–802.

70. Puggina A, Broumas A, Ricciardi W, et al. Cost-
effectiveness of screening for lung cancer with
low-dose computed tomography: a systematic literature review. Eur J Public Health 2016;26:168–75.

71. Criss SD, Cao P, Bastani M, et al. Cost-Effectiveness
Analysis of Lung Cancer Screening in the United
States: A Comparative Modeling Study. Ann Intern
Med 2019;171:796–804.

72. Kowada A. Cost-effectiveness and health impact of
lung cancer screening with low-dose computed tomography for never smokers in Japan and the
United States: a modelling study. BMC Pulm Med
2022;22(1):19.

73. Hammer MM, Eckel AL, Palazzo LL, et al. Cost-
effectiveness of treatment thresholds for subsolid
pulmonary nodules in CT lung cancer screening.
Radiology 2021;300:586–93.

74. Goehler A, McMahon PM, Lumish HS, et al. Cost-
effectiveness of follow-up of pulmonary nodules incidentally detected on cardiac computed tomographic angiography in patients with suspected
coronary artery disease. Circulation 2014;130:
668–75.

75. Gilbert CR, Ely R, Fathi JT, et al. The economic impact
of a nurse practitioner-directed lung cancer screening,
incidental pulmonary nodule, and tobacco-cessation
clinic. JTCVS 2018;155(1):416–22.

76. Clinical Preventive Service Recommendation: Lung
Cancer. American Academy of Family Physicians
(AAFP), 2013. Available at: https://www.aafp.org/
patient-care/clinical-recommendations/all/lung-cancer.
html. Accessed January 19, 2023.

77. Ersek JL, Eberth JM, McDonnell KK, et al. Knowledge of, attitudes toward, and use of low-dose
computed tomography for lung cancer screening
among family physicians. Cancer 2016;122:
2324–31.

78. Santo L., Okeyode T., National Ambulatory Medical
Care Survey: 2018 National Summary Tables.
Available at: https://www.cdc.gov/nchs/data/ahcd/
namcs_summary/2018-namcs-web-tables-508.pdf.
Accessed January 19, 2023.

79. Clinical Preventive Service Recommendation: Lung
Cancer. American Academy of Family Physicians
(AAFP). 2021. Available at: https://www.aafp.org/
family-physician/patient-care/clinical-
recommendations/all-clinical-recommendations/lung-
cancer.html. Accessed January 19, 2023.

Update on Lung Cancer Screening Guideline

Priyanka Senthil, BS, Sangkavi Kuhan, BS, Alexandra L. Potter, BS, Chi-Fu Jeffrey Yang, MD*

KEYWORDS

- Lung cancer screening • Cancer screening eligibility • Computed tomography • Early detection
- Disparities • Risk prediction • Risk assessment • USPSTF

KEY POINTS

- Lung cancer screening using low-dose computed tomography is an evidence-based approach to reduce lung cancer mortality.
- About 14.5 million people are eligible for lung cancer screening in the United States but less than 6% of high-risk individuals are currently being screened.
- Although the updated 2021 United States Preventive Services Task Force (USPSTF) lung cancer screening guideline expands screening eligibility, many people at risk for lung cancer continue to be ineligible.
- Racial/ethnic and sex disparities in lung cancer screening continue to persist and, in some cases, are widened under the revised 2021 USPSTF lung cancer screening guideline.
- Lung cancer risk prediction models, biomarkers, and deep learning may help to reduce disparities in lung cancer screening.

INTRODUCTION

Lung cancer screening using low-dose computed tomography (LDCT) is an evidence-based approach that has been shown to reduce lung cancer mortality in two large randomized controlled trials,[1,2] and it is currently recommended for individuals meeting requisite age and smoking history criteria.[3]

This review provides a background on lung cancer screening, evaluates the effect of recent changes in the lung cancer screening guideline, analyzes the successes and limitations of the current guideline, and considers future directions.

OVERVIEW OF THE STATUS OF LUNG CANCER SCREENING IN THE UNITED STATES
Introduction of Lung Cancer Screening

In the 1970s, many early clinical trials in the field of lung cancer investigated the use of sputum cytology and chest radiography as potential methods for lung cancer screening.[4] However, no strong evidence was found to support the use of either method. Research on lung cancer screening slowed until the 1990s when the first clinical trial evaluating the mortality benefit of LDCT took place, led by investigators in Japan.[5] The Early Lung Cancer Action Project, led by investigators in North America,[6] quickly followed, along with numerous other studies in the United States, Japan, and Europe that found reduced lung cancer mortality with lung cancer screening through LDCT. However, in 2004, the United States Preventive Services Task Force (USPSTF) released a statement that evidence was insufficient to recommend for or against lung cancer screening by any method.[7]

The USPSTF first recommended lung cancer screening in 2013, following the growing evidence of the benefit of LDCT from other significant studies that took place during that time, in particular, the National Lung Screening Trial (NLST).[1] The USPSTF recommended annual LDCT screening for lung cancer in adults aged 55 to 80 years who had a 30 pack-year cigarette smoking

Division of Thoracic Surgery, Massachusetts General Hospital, 55 Fruit Street, Boston, MA 02114, USA
* Corresponding author.
E-mail address: cjyang@mgh.harvard.edu

Thorac Surg Clin 33 (2023) 323–331
https://doi.org/10.1016/j.thorsurg.2023.04.002
1547-4127/23/© 2023 Elsevier Inc. All rights reserved.

history or more and who were currently smoking or had quit smoking within the past 15 years (Grade B recommendation).[7]

Early Impact of the 2013 United States Preventive Services Task Force Lung Cancer Screening Guideline

The introduction of the 2013 lung cancer screening guideline coincided with improvements in the early diagnosis of lung cancer and survival at a population level. From 2014 to 2018, the percentage of stage I non-small cell lung cancer (NSCLC) cases among patients aged 55 to 80 years increased by 3.9% per year (30.2% to 35.5%), whereas no significant increase was observed from 2010 to 2013 (27.8% to 29.4%).[8] Similarly, from 2014 to 2018, the median all-cause survival of patients aged 55 to 80 years increased at a yearly rate of 11.9% (from 19.7 to 28.2 months), almost 3 times higher than in 2010 to 2013.[8] It is estimated that 10,000 lives were saved because of the increase in the early detection of localized lung cancers in the United States from 2014 to 2018.[8]

Limitations of the 2013 United States Preventive Services Task Force Screening Guideline

Although the introduction of a national lung cancer screening guideline was a major step forward, the guideline had several notable limitations.

RACIAL DISPARITIES

The 2013 screening guideline was heavily based on the results of the NLST trial, in which the majority of participants were white (NLST: 91% white, <5% Black, and <2% Hispanic or Latino).[1] Given that the epidemiology of lung cancer varies across racial and ethnic groups, the 2013 lung cancer screening guideline may not have been appropriately suited for racial minorities. For example, studies have reported that Black,[9] Indigenous/Native,[10] and Hispanic[11] individuals are more likely to be diagnosed with lung cancer at younger ages than non-Hispanic white individuals.

Using the Black Women's Health Study (BWHS), one study evaluated the proportion of Black women diagnosed with lung cancer who would have been eligible for screening under the 2013 USPSTF guideline. The study found that only 22.7% of BWHS participants with lung cancer would have been eligible for screening, suggesting that the 2013 guideline would have missed many Black women at high risk for lung cancer.[12]

SEX DISPARITIES

Women diagnosed with lung cancer are more likely to have not smoked or smoke fewer cigarettes per day than men, oftentimes falling short of the 20 pack-year smoking requirement for lung cancer screening.[13] Women are also more likely to be diagnosed with lung cancer at younger ages and may not meet the minimum age criteria required for screening eligibility.[13,14] Screening criteria that optimize the smoking history and age requirements for men and women separately may be more efficacious.

CATEGORICAL AGE AND SMOKING RESTRICTIONS

Under the updated guideline, individuals who quit smoking more than 15 years ago continue to be ineligible for lung cancer screening. This is a significant concern because up to 45.7% of lung cancers that occur in individuals who have formerly smoked occur more than 15 years after quitting smoking.[15]

Furthermore, individuals aged older than 80 years would be ineligible to undergo screening. With the increasing life expectancy of Americans, and advancements in treatments such as minimally invasive surgery and stereotactic body radiotherapy, older patients may benefit from screening because they may still be able to undergo treatment of lung cancer.

UPDATED 2021 UNITED STATES PREVENTIVE SERVICES TASK FORCE LUNG CANCER SCREENING GUIDELINE

In March 2021, the USPSTF revised its guideline based on more recently published studies and statistical modeling. Annual lung cancer screening is now recommended among adults aged 50 to 80 years with a 20 pack-year smoking history or more and who currently smoke or have quit smoking within the past 15 years (Grade B recommendation).[3]

SUCCESSES OF THE 2021 UNITED STATES PREVENTIVE SERVICES TASK FORCE LUNG CANCER SCREENING GUIDELINE

The new USPSTF screening guideline brings two greatly welcomed changes by lowering the minimum age and smoking history requirements for screening.

The revised screening guideline increases screening eligibility, particularly among women and racial minorities who often have lower smoking histories than their male and white counterparts, respectively.[13] Furthermore, it is known that racial minorities develop lung cancer at a younger age than their white counterparts; therefore, lowering the minimum age threshold for screening may increase the proportion of lung cancers caught at an early stage among patients from racial and ethnic minority groups.[16,17] Under the new criteria, an estimated 14.5 million Americans will be eligible for screening, up from 8 million Americans under the 2013 criteria.[17]

Modeling studies show that the updated guideline reduces lung cancer mortality by 13.0% compared to 9.8% with the 2013 guideline.[18] Moreover, the proportion of non-Hispanic Black individuals eligible for lung cancer screening is predicted to have increased from 1.9% to 3.9% with the revised criteria.[3] This marks a 107% increase in the relative proportion of non-Hispanic Black adults who are eligible for lung cancer screening.

One study assessed the screening eligibility of Black women diagnosed with lung cancer in the BWHS according to the 2021 guideline. The researchers found that the revised guideline led to approximately a 50% increase in lung cancer screening eligibility; 22.7% of BWHS participants with lung cancer would have been eligible for lung cancer screening under the 2013 guideline, whereas that proportion increased to 33.9% under the 2021 guideline.[12]

According to a cross-sectional study that looked at respondents to the Behavioral Risk Factor Surveillance System from 2017 to 2018 who met the revised USPSTF screening guideline, screening eligibility among individuals who currently smoked or formerly smoked increased by 30.3% in men, 40.5% in women and 31.9% in white, 76.7% in Black, and 78.1% in Hispanic populations.[19]

LIMITATIONS OF THE 2021 UNITED STATES PREVENTIVE SERVICES TASK FORCE LUNG CANCER SCREENING GUIDELINE
Persistent Racial and Sex Disparities

Even under the 2021 lung cancer screening guideline, there is a lower odds of screening eligibility for women compared with men and for Black and Hispanic individuals compared with white individuals.[19]

Looking at the BWHS, out of 314 patients with lung cancer who smoked, 67.8% did not meet screening eligibility under the 2021 guideline due to a smoking history of less than 20 pack-years, and 46.2% were deemed ineligible for screening because they had quit smoking more than 15 years prior.[12] Sixty-six percent of the patients with lung cancer still would have been ineligible for screening.[12]

In the Multiethnic Cohort, 43.3% of lung cancer cases were eligible for screening under the 2021 USPSTF screening criteria compared with 35.1% of lung cancer cases under the 2013 USPSTF criteria.[20] However, the findings of the Multiethnic Cohort suggest that screening disparities persist among women and racial/ethnic minority populations.[20] Within the 2021 USPSTF screening criteria, the primary reason for screening ineligibility was the quit-years criterion, with 71.2% of ineligible white and 70.3% of ineligible Japanese American patients exceeding the 15 quit-year threshold.[20] The second most common reason for ineligibility was the 20 pack-year criterion, with 70.0% of ineligible Black and 65.7% of ineligible Latino patients having a smoking history below this threshold.[20]

Although the revised USPSTF guideline may increase lung cancer screening eligibility at a population level, screening inequalities among racial/ethnic minorities and women will remain unless the eligibility criteria are reviewed, tailored, and improved.

High-Risk Populations are Ineligible

Certain populations are known to be at high-risk for lung cancer but continue to be excluded from the screening criteria.

Human Immunodeficiency Virus

Lung cancer is the leading cause of cancer-related deaths in people with HIV, and lung cancer incidence has been consistently reported as being higher in people with HIV than the general population.[21–26] The current USPSTF lung cancer screening guideline also performs poorly in people living with HIV. People with HIV are younger (mean age 56.8 vs 68.0 years, $P = .014$) and are more likely to present with advanced disease at diagnosis (68% vs 49%, $P < .001$) compared with patients without HIV.[27] This is not only due to the higher rates of smoking[25,28,29] in patients with HIV but also due to independent factors specifically associated with HIV infection that contribute to this increased risk.[25,26,30–33]

A study that conducted retrospective analysis of patients with HIV with and without lung cancer in the Women's Interagency HIV Study and the Multicenter AIDS Cohort Study concluded that in order to optimize screening criteria for women with HIV and achieve a sensitivity of 52% and specificity of 75%, the criteria should include women aged 49 years or older with a smoking history of 16 pack-years or greater and a quit time of 15 years or less.[34] For men with HIV, to achieve 82% sensitivity and 76% specificity, the screening criteria should include men aged 43 years or older with a smoking history of greater than 19 pack-years and a quit time of 15 years or less.[34]

Prior Cancer Survivors

Prior cancer survivors are at a higher risk of developing a primary lung cancer than the general population.

A study evaluating patients diagnosed with one of the 10 most prevalent cancers (prostate, breast, lung, colon, rectum, bladder, uterus, kidney, melanoma, and non-Hodgkin lymphoma) between 1992 and 2008 from the Surveillance, Epidemiology, and End Results database found that around 1 in 12 patients diagnosed with a common cancer were later diagnosed with a second malignancy, the most common being lung cancer.[35] Lung cancer represented 18% of all second primary malignancies and was most common among patients with primary bladder cancer, making up one-fourth of second malignancies in this group.[35] Therefore, patients with a previous cancer diagnosis and with other risk factors for lung cancer may benefit from lung cancer screening even if they do not have a heavy smoking history or are not within the age threshold of the current USPSTF screening criteria.

Lack of Consideration of Other Risk Factors for Lung Cancer

A major limitation of the current 2021 USPSTF screening guideline is that it does not consider several well-established risk factors for lung cancer, such as exposure to radon, asbestos, and secondhand smoke, air pollution, inflammatory lung diseases, and a family history of lung cancer. Radon is the second leading cause of lung cancer after smoking and the leading cause of lung cancer in individuals who do not smoke.[36] Individuals living in areas with high levels of radon and asbestos might be at increased risk of lung cancer. Furthermore, veterans,[37] firefighters,[38] construction workers,[39] and individuals in other occupations that result in extended exposure to such environmental carcinogens may be at elevated risk for lung cancer. Therefore, the current screening criteria may miss a large proportion of patients at high-risk for lung cancer who might have no or light smoking histories.

The Taiwan Lung Cancer Screening for Never Smoker Trial (TALENT) study, a national lung cancer screening study conducted in Taiwan, enrolled 12,011 participants, almost all of whom (93.3%) had no smoking history.[40] Surprisingly, the incidence of lung cancer was 2.6%,[40] which is notably higher than the rates reported in the NLST and Nederlands–Leuvens Longkanker Screenings Onderzoek (NELSON) trials (1.1% and 0.9%, respectively).[1,2]

The eligibility criteria for the TALENT study included individuals who did not smoke or smoked less than 10 pack-years and had quit smoking for more than 15 years, were between the ages of 55 and 75 years, had a normal chest radiograph, and had at least one of the following risk factors for lung cancer: a history of lung cancer in the family in first-degree, second-degree, or third-degree relatives; exposure to secondhand smoke; an earlier diagnosis of tuberculosis or chronic obstructive pulmonary disease (COPD); and cooking without ventilation or a cooking index 110 or greater (regular exposure to frying food).[40] Almost three-fourths of the participants were women and one-half of the participants had a family history of lung cancer.[40]

Of the 12,011 scans performed, 2094 (17.4%) were considered abnormal.[40] Lung cancer was diagnosed in 311 subjects (2.6%) and 254 subjects (2.1%) had invasive lung cancer. About 96.5% of diagnosed cancers were stage 0 or stage I.[40] In subjects with a family history of lung cancer, the prevalence of lung cancer and invasive lung cancer was 3.2% and 2.6%, respectively, compared with 2.0% and 1.6% in those without a family history.[40]

The results of the TALENT study suggest that lung cancer screening may be beneficial in individuals with non-smoking-related risk factors for lung cancer, even in the absence of a heavy smoking history.

POTENTIAL SOLUTIONS TO THE LIMITATIONS OF THE CURRENT SCREENING ELIGIBILITY CRITERIA
Risk-Prediction Models

Multivariable mathematical models estimate a person's lung cancer risk during a period of several years using risk factors beyond age and smoking history.

One of the most well-validated risk-prediction models is the PLCOm2012[41,42] (a logistic regression model) that was constructed to forecast the 6-year risk of lung cancer in ever-smoking participants of the Prostate, Lung, Colorectal, and Ovarian Cancer Screening Trial.[43–51] It includes variables such as age, race or ethnicity, education, body mass index, COPD, personal history of cancer, family history of lung cancer, smoking status, smoking duration, smoking intensity (cigarettes per day), and years since smoking cessation.[42]

A previous study showed that risk-based screening using the PLCOm2012 model with a risk threshold of 1.51% improved sensitivity to 75.7% compared with 43.3% with the 2021 USPSTF criteria, and this increase was observed across all racial and ethnic groups, with a range of 17.2% to 39.6%.[20]

Several studies have suggested that the PLCOm2012 model reduces racial and ethnic disparities in screening eligibility when compared with either the 2013[52] or the 2021[53] USPSTF screening criteria. However, these conclusions are mainly drawn from analyses conducted on disparities among Black patients.[53] Using the PLCOm2012 model, risk-based screening reduced racial and ethnic disparities in screening among Black individuals from 11.2% to 5.1% but widened screening disparities for Japanese Americans (from 9.6% to 12.8%) and Latinos (from 12.4% to 28.6%).[20]

The PLCOm2012 model is promising because it may help refine the selection of high-risk individuals with a remote history of smoking (ie, those who quit more than 15 years ago) and with lighter smoking histories (ie, those who have fewer than 20 pack-years) for lung cancer screening. The current model increases sensitivity and reduces racial and ethnic disparities among Black patients but will need to be adjusted to better address screening disparities in other racial groups.

There are other risk prediction models such as the Bach,[54] Liverpool Lung Project (LLP),[55] Two-Stage Clonal Expansion (TSCE) models for incidence and death,[56–58] Knoke,[59] and simplified PLCOm2012 and LLP[60]] models. These risk-prediction models were evaluated by Ten Haaf and colleagues[43] in both the NLST and PLCO cohorts. The results highlighted that when each model was set to its specific threshold, all had a higher sensitivities and specificities when compared with the NLST criteria, which had a specificity of 62.2% and sensitivity of 71.4%.[43] The PLCOm2012, Bach, and TSCE incidence performed the best with specificities greater than 62.3% and sensitivities greater than 79.8%.[43]

Despite retrospective studies that have shown that risk-prediction models greatly reduce racial disparities, the United States is one of several countries to continue using risk criteria instead of risk-prediction models.

Biomarkers and Deep Learning Models

Molecular biomarkers can refine patient selection for lung cancer screening and improve risk-stratification.[61] The EarlyCDT-Lung test, which measures autoantibodies relating to lung cancer-associated antigens, has been shown to predict lung cancer risk with a specificity of 91% and sensitivity of 37% to 41%.[62,63] Other biomarkers that can be used as adjuncts for lung cancer screening include complement fragments, DNA methylation, miR-NAs, protein profiling, and exhaled breath condensate.[64] Biomarker testing may benefit minority populations with high incidences of lung cancer among individuals without a significant smoking history.

Several deep learning (DL) algorithms have been developed to detect and characterize lung nodules from chest radiographs or LDCTs. For example, Sybil uses a single LDCT scan to predict lung cancers occurring up to 6 years after a scan.[65] Sybil was able to predict lung cancer within one year with an area under the curve of 0.86 to 0.94 on three independent datasets.[65] However, there must be an increase in the evidence of long-term outcomes of using DL models in clinical practice.[66] Other articles cover the utility of biomarkers and DL in greater depth.

SUMMARY AND DISCUSSION

Although the expansion of the USPSTF criteria has increased lung cancer screening eligibility among the general population, racial/ethnic minority groups and women are still less likely to be eligible for screening because they tend to have lighter smoking histories and are more likely to be diagnosed with lung cancer at younger ages. Furthermore, the current criteria do not consider non-smoking-related risk factors such as a history of HIV and COPD, family history of lung cancer, and exposure to radon and asbestos.

However, drastically liberalizing the lung cancer screening criteria is not the solution as it may result in higher rates of false-positive tests and overdiagnosis, unnecessary radiation exposure, and excessive follow-up testing for patients who truly are not at high risk for lung cancer. It is crucial that the screening criteria only target patients at high risk for lung cancer to ensure the benefits of screening outweigh any potential harms.

Under the current structure, the USPSTF aims to review its recommendations every 5 years for either an update or reaffirmation, projecting 2026 as the year for potentially revised lung cancer screening criteria. Some have recommended removing the 15 quit-year threshold; one study found that doing so would increase the proportion of Black women eligible for screening from 33.9% to 48.2%.[12] There is also debate on whether to remove the upper age limit for screening and quit-year threshold to mirror the National Comprehensive Cancer Network's lung cancer screening guideline, which recommends screening for any individual aged 50 years or older with 20 pack-years or more of smoking history.

The use of lung cancer risk prediction models to supplement categorical screening criteria may be one strategy to improve the selection of high-risk individuals for screening across all populations. The strength of risk prediction models is the ability to expand criteria while still targeting only high-risk patients. Risk prediction models that account for significant non-smoking-related risk factors can increase screening eligibility among high-risk populations without a heavy smoking history. Additionally, the incorporation of factors such as race and sex into risk models can help reduce inequities in eligibility. The use of lung cancer risk prediction models may also inform screening intervals.

However, optimizing lung cancer screening criteria is only half of the battle in achieving equity in lung cancer screening for all high-risk populations. The other half involves raising awareness of and access to screening. Currently, only 5.8% of eligible Americans are getting screened for lung cancer. There are several factors that are contributing to this staggeringly low uptake of screening. The primary factor is the lack of awareness about screening among the general public.

Lung cancer screening awareness remains low among Americans. According to one study involving 240 participants, 56% of participants did not know about screening for lung cancer and 65% were unaware that LDCT screening was the appropriate test.[67] Although familiarity with lung cancer screening is low, more people are willing to undergo screening if it is recommended by their primary care physicians (PCPs).[67,68] However, studies reveal that not all PCPs are aware of the lung cancer screening recommendations.[69] Continuing medical education programs surrounding lung cancer screening may be able to address these gaps.

Moreover, there are numerous barriers to lung cancer screening including cost, access to nearby screening centers, and stigma.[70] The implementation of routine lung cancer screening reminders for patients needing annual scans, integration of nurse navigators to aid patients in the process of scheduling and receiving a scan, assistance programs to cover transportation costs, and the introduction of mobile screening vans in rural geographic locations are potential solutions that have shown to increase the uptake of lung cancer screening.

Importance of Community Outreach to Increase Screening Awareness

Looking ahead, increasing lung cancer screening eligibility and awareness of early detection is important and must be a priority. One organization spearheading lung cancer awareness and advocacy is the American Lung Cancer Screening Initiative (ALCSI).

ALCSI worked with US Congress members and senators to draft and advocate for the first-ever US House and Senate resolutions recognizing the importance of the early-detection of lung cancer through screening. In December 2022, the US Senate passed a bipartisan resolution (S.Res.863) for the third year in a row designating November 2022 as National Lung Cancer Awareness Month and expressing support for the early detection and treatment of lung cancer. S.Res.863 expands on the previous resolutions, S.Res.780 and S.Res.462, by emphasizing the need for efforts to increase awareness of screening among Veterans, women, and racial minorities. The resolutions were passed by unanimous consent by all 100 senators.

ALCSI has worked with mayors and governors from all 50 US states and Canada to issue more than 345 proclamations recognizing November as National Lung Cancer Awareness Month. Furthermore, ALCSI has worked with numerous state leaders to share public service announcements about lung cancer screening in local communities. Engaging trusted community leaders in awareness efforts has been an effective method to reach different populations.

ALCSI's 30+ college chapters hold canvassing and tabling events, presentations, White Ribbon builds, and fundraisers to teach community members of all age groups, backgrounds, cultures, and identities about the importance of lung cancer screening and early detection, reaching more than 10,000 people. Attendees are encouraged to take ALCSI's lung cancer screening eligibility assessment, which identifies individuals eligible for lung cancer screening and helps them connect to local screening centers. Through these activities, ALCSI is pushing the momentum forward on increasing screening engagement among high-risk individuals across the United States.

With the goal of getting lung cancer screening information in front of more eyes, ALCSI also started a +1 campaign. Instead of approaching community members with the question "Are you eligible for lung cancer screening," ALCSI asks "Do you know someone eligible for lung cancer screening." Rephrasing the question in this manner makes outreach applicable to anyone and taps into the networks and connections of each individual.

In order to reduce disparities in lung cancer, it is critical to acknowledge and address disparities in lung cancer screening eligibility and access. Mounting evidence is showing that the current 2021 USPSTF screening criteria have limitations, inadvertently excluding patients who might be at high-risk for lung cancer but who do not meet requisite age or smoking history criteria. The lung cancer screening guideline must be revised to address the ever-prevalent inequities in screening, and advocacy and awareness efforts must be parallelly driven to increase access to screening.

CLINICS CARE POINTS

- Several randomized controlled studies have shown that LDCT screening can identify lung cancers at earlier stages and reduce lung cancer mortality when compared with no screening or screening with chest radiography.
- The revised 2021 USPSTF lung cancer screening guideline expands lung cancer screening eligibility to individuals aged 50 to 80 years, who have a 20 pack-year smoking history or more, and who currently smoke or quit within the last 15 years.
- Under the 2021 USPSTF lung cancer screening guideline, 14.5 million people are estimated to be eligible for lung cancer screening in the United States.
- However, less than 6% of high-risk Americans are currently being screened for lung cancer due to a lack of awareness among the public and among health-care providers, as well as barriers to lung cancer screening, such as cost, distance, and stigma.
- Racial minorities and women with lung cancer are more likely to be diagnosed at younger ages and to have lighter smoking histories.
- There are other risk factors for lung cancer such as a family history of lung cancer, a personal history of chronic lung diseases, and exposure to radon, asbestos, and secondhand smoke that are not currently accounted for in the 2021 USPSTF lung cancer screening guideline.
- The use of lung cancer risk prediction models, biomarkers, and deep learning may help to refine the selection of patients at high-risk for lung cancer and reduce disparities in lung cancer screening eligibility.

DISCLOSURE

P. Senthil, S. Kuhan, A.L. Potter, C.J. Yang have unpaid leadership roles in the American Lung Cancer Screening Initiative (a 501(c)(3) non-profit). No other disclosures were reported.

REFERENCES

1. Aberle DR, Adams AM, Berg CD, et al. Reduced lung-cancer mortality with low-dose computed tomographic screening. N Engl J Med 2011;365(5):395–409.
2. de Koning HJ, van der Aalst CM, de Jong PA, et al. Reduced Lung-Cancer Mortality with Volume CT Screening in a Randomized Trial. N Engl J Med 2020;382(6):503–13.
3. Krist AH, Davidson KW, Mangione CM, et al. Screening for Lung Cancer: US Preventive Services Task Force Recommendation Statement. JAMA 2021;325(10):962–70.
4. Marcus PM, Bergstralh EJ, Fagerstrom RM, et al. Lung cancer mortality in the Mayo Lung Project: impact of extended follow-up. J Natl Cancer Inst 2000;92(16):1308–16.
5. Kaneko M, Eguchi K, Ohmatsu H, et al. Peripheral lung cancer: screening and detection with low-dose spiral CT versus radiography. Radiology 1996;201(3):798–802.
6. Henschke CI, McCauley DI, Yankelevitz DF, et al. Early Lung Cancer Action Project: overall design and findings from baseline screening. Lancet 1999;354(9173):99–105.
7. Moyer VA, Force USPST. Screening for lung cancer: U.S. Preventive Services Task Force recommendation statement. Ann Intern Med 2014;160(5):330–8.
8. Potter AL, Rosenstein AL, Kiang MV, et al. Association of computed tomography screening with lung cancer stage shift and survival in the United States: quasi-experimental study. BMJ 2022;376:e069008.
9. Shusted CS, Evans NR, Juon HS, et al. Association of Race With Lung Cancer Risk Among Adults Undergoing Lung Cancer Screening. JAMA Netw Open 2021;4(4):e214509.
10. Borondy Kitts AK. The Patient Perspective on Lung Cancer Screening and Health Disparities. J Am Coll Radiol 2019;16(4 Pt B):601–6.
11. Parada H, Vu AH, Pinheiro PS, et al. Comparing Age at Cancer Diagnosis between Hispanics and Non-Hispanic Whites in the United States. Cancer Epidemiol Biomarkers Prev 2021;30(10):1904–12.
12. Potter AL, Yang CJ, Woolpert KM, et al. Evaluating Eligibility of US Black Women Under USPSTF Lung Cancer Screening Guidelines. JAMA Oncol 2022;8(1):163–4.
13. Fidler-Benaoudia MM, Torre LA, Bray F, et al. Lung cancer incidence in young women vs. young men: A systematic analysis in 40 countries. Int J Cancer 2020;147(3):811–9.
14. Jemal A, Miller KD, Ma J, et al. Higher Lung Cancer Incidence in Young Women Than Young Men in the United States. N Engl J Med 2018;378(21):1999–2009.

15. Pinsky PF, Zhu CS, Kramer BS. Lung cancer risk by years since quitting in 30+ pack year smokers. J Med Screen 2015;22(3):151–7.

16. Robbins HA, Engels EA, Pfeiffer RM, et al. Age at cancer diagnosis for blacks compared with whites in the United States. J Natl Cancer Inst 2015;107(3). https://doi.org/10.1093/jnci/dju489.

17. Landy R, Young CD, Skarzynski M, et al. Using Prediction Models to Reduce Persistent Racial and Ethnic Disparities in the Draft 2020 USPSTF Lung Cancer Screening Guidelines. J Natl Cancer Inst 2021;113(11):1590–4.

18. Meza R, Jeon J, Toumazis I, et al. Evaluation of the Benefits and Harms of Lung Cancer Screening With Low-Dose Computed Tomography: Modeling Study for the US Preventive Services Task Force. JAMA 2021;325(10):988–97.

19. Reese TJ, Schlechter CR, Potter LN, et al. Evaluation of Revised US Preventive Services Task Force Lung Cancer Screening Guideline Among Women and Racial/Ethnic Minority Populations. JAMA Netw Open 2021;4(1):e2033769.

20. Aredo JV, Choi E, Ding VY, et al. Racial and Ethnic Disparities in Lung Cancer Screening by the 2021 USPSTF Guidelines Versus Risk-Based Criteria: The Multiethnic Cohort Study. JNCI Cancer Spectr 2022;6(3). https://doi.org/10.1093/jncics/pkac033.

21. Sigel K, Makinson A, Thaler J. Lung cancer in persons with HIV. Curr Opin HIV AIDS 2017;12(1):31–8.

22. Shiels MS, Pfeiffer RM, Gail MH, et al. Cancer burden in the HIV-infected population in the United States. J Natl Cancer Inst 2011;103(9):753–62.

23. Winstone TA, Man SFP, Hull M, et al. Epidemic of lung cancer in patients with HIV infection. Chest 2013;143(2):305–14.

24. Morlat P, Roussillon C, Henard S, et al. Causes of death among HIV-infected patients in France in 2010 (national survey): trends since 2000. AIDS 2014;28(8):1181–91.

25. Sigel K, Wisnivesky J, Gordon K, et al. HIV as an independent risk factor for incident lung cancer. AIDS 2012;26(8):1017–25.

26. Hessol NA, Martínez-Maza O, Levine AM, et al. Lung cancer incidence and survival among HIV-infected and uninfected women and men. AIDS 2015;29(10):1183–93.

27. Galeas JN, Grossberg RM, Serrano M, et al. Improving lung cancer screening in the HIV population. J Clin Oncol 2019;37(27_suppl):69.

28. Park LS, Hernández-Ramírez RU, Silverberg MJ, et al. Prevalence of non-HIV cancer risk factors in persons living with HIV/AIDS: a meta-analysis. AIDS 2016;30(2):273–91.

29. Clifford GM, Lise M, Franceschi S, et al. Lung cancer in the Swiss HIV Cohort Study: role of smoking, immunodeficiency and pulmonary infection. Br J Cancer 2012;106(3):447–52.

30. Shiels MS, Cole SR, Mehta SH, et al. Lung cancer incidence and mortality among HIV-infected and HIV-uninfected injection drug users. J Acquir Immune Defic Syndr 2010;55(4):510–5.

31. Kirk GD, Merlo C, O' Driscoll P, et al. HIV infection is associated with an increased risk for lung cancer, independent of smoking. Clin Infect Dis 2007;45(1):103–10.

32. Guiguet M, Boué F, Cadranel J, et al. Effect of immunodeficiency, HIV viral load, and antiretroviral therapy on the risk of individual malignancies (FHDH-ANRS CO4): a prospective cohort study. Lancet Oncol 2009;10(12):1152–9.

33. Hleyhel M, Bouvier AM, Belot A, et al. Risk of non-AIDS-defining cancers among HIV-1-infected individuals in France between 1997 and 2009: results from a French cohort. AIDS 2014;28(14):2109–18.

34. Sellers SA, Edmonds A, Ramirez C, et al. Optimal Lung Cancer Screening Criteria Among Persons Living With HIV. J Acquir Immune Defic Syndr 2022;90(2):184–92.

35. Donin N, Filson C, Drakaki A, et al. Risk of second primary malignancies among cancer survivors in the United States, 1992 through 2008. Cancer 2016;122(19):3075–86.

36. WHO Handbook on Indoor Radon: A Public Health Perspective. World Health Organization; 2009.

37. Grier W, Abbas H, Gebeyehu RR, et al. Military exposures and lung cancer in United States veterans. Semin Oncol 2022. https://doi.org/10.1053/j.seminoncol.2022.06.010.

38. Navarro KM, Kleinman MT, Mackay CE, et al. Wildland firefighter smoke exposure and risk of lung cancer and cardiovascular disease mortality. Environ Res 2019;173:462–8.

39. Calvert GM, Luckhaupt S, Lee SJ, et al. Lung cancer risk among construction workers in California, 1988-2007. Am J Ind Med 2012;55(5):412–22.

40. Yang P. PS01. 02 national lung cancer screening program in Taiwan: the TALENT study. J Thorac Oncol 2021;16(3):S58.

41. Tammemägi MC, Church TR, Hocking WG, et al. Evaluation of the lung cancer risks at which to screen ever- and never-smokers: screening rules applied to the PLCO and NLST cohorts. PLoS Med 2014;11(12):e1001764.

42. Tammemägi MC, Katki HA, Hocking WG, et al. Selection criteria for lung-cancer screening. N Engl J Med 2013;368(8):728–36.

43. Ten Haaf K, Jeon J, Tammemägi MC, et al. Risk prediction models for selection of lung cancer screening candidates: A retrospective validation study. PLoS Med 2017;14(4):e1002277.

44. Weber M, Yap S, Goldsbury D, et al. Identifying high risk individuals for targeted lung cancer screening: Independent validation of the PLCO. Int J Cancer 2017;141(2):242–53.

45. Tammemagi MC, Schmidt H, Martel S, et al. Participant selection for lung cancer screening by risk modelling (the Pan-Canadian Early Detection of Lung Cancer [PanCan] study): a single-arm, prospective study. Lancet Oncol 2017;18(11):1523–31.

46. Li K, Hüsing A, Sookthai D, et al. Selecting High-Risk Individuals for Lung Cancer Screening: A Prospective Evaluation of Existing Risk Models and Eligibility Criteria in the German EPIC Cohort. Cancer Prev Res 2015;8(9):777–85.

47. Hüsing A, Kaaks R. Risk prediction models versus simplified selection criteria to determine eligibility for lung cancer screening: an analysis of German federal-wide survey and incidence data. Eur J Epidemiol 2020;35(10):899–912.

48. Crosbie PA, Balata H, Evison M, et al. Implementing lung cancer screening: baseline results from a community-based 'Lung Health Check' pilot in deprived areas of Manchester. Thorax 2019;74(4): 405–9.

49. Crosbie PA, Balata H, Evison M, et al. Second round results from the Manchester 'Lung Health Check' community-based targeted lung cancer screening pilot. Thorax 2019;74(7):700–4.

50. Kavanagh J, Liu G, Menezes R, et al. Importance of Long-term Low-Dose CT Follow-up after Negative Findings at Previous Lung Cancer Screening. Radiology 2018;289(1):218–24.

51. Aggarwal R, Lam ACL, McGregor M, et al. Outcomes of Long-term Interval Rescreening With Low-Dose Computed Tomography for Lung Cancer in Different Risk Cohorts. J Thorac Oncol 2019; 14(6):1003–11.

52. Han SS, Chow E, Ten Haaf K, et al. Disparities of National Lung Cancer Screening Guidelines in the US Population. J Natl Cancer Inst 2020;112(11): 1136–42.

53. Pasquinelli MM, Tammemägi MC, Kovitz KL, et al. Risk Prediction Model Versus United States Preventive Services Task Force Lung Cancer Screening Eligibility Criteria: Reducing Race Disparities. J Thorac Oncol 2020;15(11):1738–47.

54. Bach PB, Kattan MW, Thornquist MD, et al. Variations in lung cancer risk among smokers. J Natl Cancer Inst 2003;95(6):470–8.

55. Marcus MW, Chen Y, Raji OY, et al. Liverpool lung project risk prediction model for lung cancer incidence. Cancer Prev Res (Phila) 2015;8(6):570–5.

56. Hazelton W.D., Clements M.S., Moolgavkar S.H.., Multistage carcinogenesis and lung cancer mortality in three cohorts, Cancer Epidemiol Biomarkers Prev, 14 (5), 2005, 1171–1181.

57. Hazelton WD, Jeon J, Meza R, Moolgavkar SH. Chapter 8: the FHCRC lung cancer model. Risk Anal 2012;32:S99–116.

58. Meza R, Hazelton W, Colditz G, Moolgavkar S. Analysis of lung cancer incidence in the Nurses' Health and the Health Professionals' Follow-Up Studies using a multistage carcinogenesis model. Cancer Causes Control 2008;19(3):317–28.

59. Knoke JD, Burns DM, Thun MJ. The change in excess risk of lung cancer attributable to smoking following smoking cessation: an examination of different analytic approaches using CPS-I data. Cancer Causes Control 2007;19(2):207–19.

60. Cassidy A., Myles J.P., van Tongeren M., et al., The LLP risk model: an individual risk prediction model for lung cancer, Br J Cancer, 98 (2), 2008, 270–276.

61. Ramaswamy A. Lung Cancer Screening: Review and 2021 Update. Curr Pulmonol Rep 2022;11(1): 15–28.

62. Jett JR, Peek LJ, Fredericks L, et al. Audit of the autoantibody test, EarlyCDT®-lung, in 1600 patients: an evaluation of its performance in routine clinical practice. Lung Cancer 2014;83(1):51–5.

63. Chapman CJ, Healey GF, Murray A, et al. EarlyCDT®-Lung test: improved clinical utility through additional autoantibody assays. Tumour Biol 2012; 33(5):1319–26.

64. Marmor H.N., Zorn J.T., Deppen S.A., et al., Biomarkers in lung cancer screening: a narrative review, Curr Chall Thorac Surg, 5:5, 2023.

65. Mikhael PG, Wohlwend J, Yala A, et al. Sybil: A Validated Deep Learning Model to Predict Future Lung Cancer Risk From a Single Low-Dose Chest Computed Tomography. J Clin Oncol 2023;12: JCO2201345. https://doi.org/10.1200/JCO.22.01345.

66. Lee JH, Hwang EJ, Kim H, et al. A narrative review of deep learning applications in lung cancer research: from screening to prognostication. Transl Lung Cancer Res 2022;11(6):1217–29.

67. Monu J, Triplette M, Wood DE, et al. Evaluating Knowledge, Attitudes, and Beliefs About Lung Cancer Screening Using Crowdsourcing. Chest 2020; 158(1):386–92.

68. Sharma A, Kasza K, Hyland A, et al. Awareness and interest in lung cancer screening among current and former smokers: findings from the ITC United States Survey. Cancer Causes Control 2019;30(7):733–45.

69. Rajupet S, Doshi D, Wisnivesky JP, et al. Attitudes About Lung Cancer Screening: Primary Care Providers Versus Specialists. Clin Lung Cance 2017; 18(6):e417–23.

70. Lei F, Lee E. Barriers to Lung Cancer Screening With Low-Dose Computed Tomography. Oncol Nurs Forum 2019;46(2):E60–71.

Building a Lung Cancer Screening Program

Neel P. Chudgar, MD[a],*, Brendon M. Stiles, MD[b]

KEYWORDS

- Lung cancer • Screening • Navigator • Multidisciplinary care

KEY POINTS

- Building a lung cancer screening program requires multidisciplinary input from primary care providers, radiologists, pulmonologists, thoracic surgeons, oncology nurses, and facility administration.
- Critical to improving uptake of lung cancer screening (LCS) is to understand the needs of the at-risk community eligible for screening and potential barriers.
- The electronic health system can assist the administration of an LCS program, but care must be taken to ensure accurate data entry.
- An adjunctive lung nodule clinic can support follow-up of LCS results, while additionally identifying and facilitating management of incidental lung nodules identified outside of screening.
- Lung cancer screening is a dynamic process that requires continued adaptation and process refinement.

INTRODUCTION

Early detection is crucial to improve outcomes for lung cancer, which continues to be the leading cause of cancer death in both men and women. Most newly diagnosed cases continue to present with advanced disease where survival is poor. Several earlier trials had begun to generate support for lung cancer screening (LCS), but it was not until 2011 that positive randomized-controlled data were presented with the seminal publication of the National Lung Screening Trial (NLST). This study demonstrated a relative reduction in lung cancer–related mortality of 20.0% with annual low-dose computed tomography (LDCT) scan.[1] Subsequent to this, LCS was supported by the United States Preventative Services Task Force with a grade B recommendation in 2013 and coverage provided by the Centers for Medicare and Medicaid Services (CMS) shortly thereafter.

Additional evidence resulting from other large, randomized trials has continued to support the mortality benefit of LCS, including data for prolonged screening following the index scan.[2,3] Despite this well-demonstrated survival advantage afforded by LCS in eligible patients, rates of uptake are poor with less than 5% of eligible patients participating.[4] Socioeconomically disadvantaged populations along with patients of color, who are at higher risk of death due to lung cancer, are at particular risk of underscreening.[5]

Reasons for low screening rates can be related to systemic, provider-, and patient-related factors. LCS, in practice now for nearly a decade, is still in its infancy relative to more established screening recommendations for other cancers. Screening for breast cancer by mammography has enjoyed support for more than 40 years, whereas colonoscopy has similarly long been accepted for colorectal cancer screening. With its more recent adoption, a lack of education and awareness of LCS may still plague medical providers.[6] The ability to integrate screening practices into existing treatment infrastructures also requires coordination and time.

[a] Montefiore Medical Center at the Albert Einstein College of Medicine, Bronx, NY, USA; [b] Division of Thoracic Surgery and Surgical Oncology, Montefiore Medical Center at the Albert Einstein College of Medicine
* Corresponding author. 3400 Bainbridge Avenue, Bronx, NY 10467.
E-mail address: nchudgar@montefiore.org

Thorac Surg Clin 33 (2023) 333–341
https://doi.org/10.1016/j.thorsurg.2023.04.008
1547-4127/23/© 2023 Elsevier Inc. All rights reserved.

Many additional barriers exist posing difficulties for more widespread adoption of LCS. Cigarette smoking remains stigmatized and has been identified as a deterrent to screening. Current smokers are less likely to adhere to LCS than former smokers, as concerns for undesirable findings and ambivalence about smoking cessation may exist.[7,8] Especially among socially disadvantaged patients who smoke, where lung cancer risk may be higher, data have demonstrated higher rates of fatalism or the belief that cancer is up to fate and that outcomes are out of one's control.[9] Medical mistrust similarly plays a role, as patients may be apprehensive about radiation risks or subsequent treatment and follow-up related to results of LCS.

Several considerations should be accounted for to build an effective and successful program for LCS. Many elements required for implementation have been identified. Although not inclusive, these include incorporation of multidisciplinary input, delineation of a discrete and efficient workflow, anticipation and management of barriers to screening uptake, and continued programmatic review and quality improvement.[10]

Perhaps most importantly, the specialized needs of the local target population must be identified such that programs can be customized to improve uptake and adherence. A one-size-fits-all approach may not apply to all patient groups. Here, we present a summary of how to build and adapt a centralized program based on our own experiences in a majority-minority population with above-average smoking rates, where the adoption of appropriate LCS has been historically challenging.

ELEMENTS FOR INCORPORATION INTO A LUNG CANCER SCREENING PROGRAM

Through the evolution of our LCS program, we have noted an important interplay between the patients we serve, the providers who refer them, and the system that completes their screening. Several elements are required for consideration to create a sustainable system. A programmatic approach to building a successful LCS program must also incorporate patient and provider perspectives in the context of the community-at-large to ensure accessibility.

Determination of Program Type

Although the subsequent focus is on the establishment of a primarily centralized screening program, determination of program type is important and requires assessment of resources available within the patient population. Centralized programs are administered by a discrete team of providers and coordinators. There is an infrastructure of shared resources that generally supports the entire process from referral to result reporting and follow-up. Decentralized programs are typically administered by individual providers who then refer patients for further care as necessary. Data have demonstrated that adherence rates for LCS are routinely higher in centralized settings, at least partially owing to the dedication of resources specifically for the purpose of screening.[11,12] Other components underlying these benefits are not fully understood yet, however, and may to some extent address disparities of care.[13] Despite this advantage, the establishment of centralized programs requires adequate time, organization, and programmatic support that may not be available or practical in all settings. Hybrid programs seek to bridge both sides where some common resources are available and may facilitate broader patient reach. Clearly, several factors must be considered in identifying the best-fit program for a patient base.

Establishing a Multidisciplinary Team

LCS benefits from multidisciplinary input that includes representation from medical providers, administrators, and nursing staff.[6,10,14] Physicians from thoracic surgery, pulmonology, and radiology can provide the needed medical oversight such that patients can undergo screening with appropriate follow-up of findings. Perhaps overlooked, however, is the role that primary care physicians (PCPs) also play in bringing eligible candidates in for screening.

PCPs can serve as the gatekeepers for LCS. However, several barriers also exist from the provider perspective that may limit referral for LDCT. With its relative novelty, some may be unaware of the eligibility criteria.[6,15,16] Recent changes to these criteria with reduced pack-year smoking requirement and a lower age cut-off may also confound knowledge for screening eligibility. Outside of knowledge constraints, time limitations may also preclude referrals for LCS.[6,17] Many elements are ultimately required to complete LCS, including verification of eligibility, shared decision-making (SDM), LDCT ordering, and result management. A centralized programmatic approach may alleviate some of the pressures on PCPs, whereby only referral is needed. By affording resources and education on eligibility to PCPs, 2 notable barriers can be addressed that may increase uptake.[6,17] In addition to providing discrete CMS-approved criteria for LCS, the primary care system should feel confident and support in a partnered screening program. We have included representatives from primary care in center-wide LCS retreats to facilitate ongoing dialogue.

Support from hospital and/or site administrators is also crucial, as LCS requires an appropriate balance of resource allocation and cost.[14,18] Several elements outside of the core providers are required for successful LCS implementation. Access to a computed tomography scanner with trained technologists, support staff, and personnel for patient scheduling and communication along with systems to track patients who have undergone screening are just a few of these needs.[19] With program expansion, reassessment of personnel and program needs to maintain efficiency is absolutely required. We recommend monthly review meetings to evaluate total referrals for LCS, timelines of referral to LDCT, and staffing metrics.

Nurse navigators have played an important role in oncology and have been used to improve several elements of lung cancer care. They facilitate access to care and data have demonstrated improved time to diagnosis and treatment when LCS is facilitated by nurse navigators.[20] Specific to LCS, nurse navigators have conducted provider education to enhance discussions surrounding tobacco cessation and support communication of results to both patients and providers.[21] Central to our LCS program is the role nurse practitioner navigators play in SDM. Advanced practice providers solely dedicated to screening thus present a valuable resource. They maintain a central role through the continuum of the screening process. By participating in a structured visit to discuss LCS, patients are afforded with a dedicated practitioner to function as a point-person for questions or concerns.

With the overall goal of identifying early-stage and potentially curable disease through LCS, surgeons and interventional pulmonologists must also have investment into screening programs.[22,23] Thoracic surgeons and interventional pulmonologists can provide an additional perspective on results of LDCT especially in the presence of lung nodules. Additive to the radiologist's interpretation, imaging results can be placed within a clinical context to further stratify nodules. With lung nodules commonly found following LDCT, surgeons and interventional pulmonologists can provide insight that may avoid unnecessary procedures and risk; alternatively, they can help expedite care for those with findings warranting intervention.[22] Multidisciplinary input and balance among team members is essential in this decision-making process. As destination care providers, surgeon assessment is particularly important in the management of screen-detected findings to ensure interventions are appropriate.[24]

Identifying Baseline Data and Population Needs

With the establishment of a multidisciplinary team, it is also important to acknowledge clinical, sociodemographic, and behavioral or cultural characteristics of the population targeted for screening. Lung cancer rates vary by region as do rates of tobacco use. Uptake of screening tends to correlate inversely with burden of lung cancer, and identifying pockets with need and high reward potential can be important for real-world implementation.[25]

Patterns of care can similarly influence how patients should be approached for entry into screening programs. Those receiving care through emergency department visits outside of primary care appointments can be difficult to capture. In underserved populations in particular, many lung cancers are diagnosed in patients without a primary care provider.[26] These patients include many patients who would otherwise be eligible for LCS. Touch points where patients may access care, such as the emergency department, can be used to identify screening candidates or reinforce the role for primary care.

In addition to logistical challenges of reaching these patients, associated sociodemographic barriers also require consideration. Black patients, who are at higher risk of lung cancer mortality than White patients, have demonstrated lower rates of LCS.[5] Owing to language barriers, Spanish-speaking Hispanic patients are similarly at risk of not receiving appropriate screening.[27] Low-income patients are also likely underscreened as are those who are uninsured.[28] Identification of these at-risk populations is critical to ensuring programmatic efforts to bring patients to care are in place.

Lastly, attitudes toward LCS can also pose a barrier and ought to be anticipated.[8] Tailored invitation strategies may be required to increase acceptance of and participation in screening, especially in disparate populations where smoking rates are high. Discussions with health care providers and potential LCS candidates within the community can inform how to optimize delivery of the program. Social media campaigns and informational events can also be subsequently designed.

As patients are identified for LCS, SDM provides another opportunity to educate patients and address potential barriers to screening. Rationale for and potential benefit of LCS can be discussed. Areas of potential anxiety, including true and false positives, need for subsequent procedures, and other incidental findings can also be addressed ahead of LDCT.[14] Smoking cessation, synergistic to screening in improving survival, can also be discussed.

Using the Electronic Health System to Create a Standardized and Reproducible Workflow

As patients are captured and referred for LCS, a standardized workflow can ensure patients are appropriately chaperoned through the screening process. Processes should be in place to confirm eligibility, perform SDM, schedule LDCT, and report results.[10,14] Although exact protocols ought to be customized to each program's population needs and resource availability, a uniform workflow can support efficiency and future scalability.

An important adjunct in the screening workflow is in use of the institutional electronic health system (EHS). The EHS can play a substantial role in facilitating LCS by providing an element of automaticity. In addition to LCS referral and eligibility assessment, the EHS has potential to communicate results and track follow-up, thus serving as the database for those enrolled.[29] However, to reap its benefits requires a baseline level of investment to optimize systems for ease of use. The system also ought to be standardized, which may pose challenges to programs that are not centralized where different referring providers may use different EHSs.[14]

A proposed role for the EHS has been to identify patients who may be eligible for LCS via age and smoking status, per USPSTF guidelines. A commonly noted bottleneck is found here, however, as inadequate or inaccurate documentation of smoking history is common.[14,30] Ensuring ease of data entry in addition to reminders during visit documentation is critical and may reinforce the importance of this element of the patient's history. Similarly, automated prompts to notify providers of screening eligibility being met on entry of patient age and smoking history may also promote referral for LCS. Until more facile and accurate documentation systems are in place, however, the EHS should not be the sole source of identifying patients for LCS.[30]

Once patients undergo LDCT, results should also be documented in templated format through the Lung Imaging Reporting and Data System (Lung-RADS). The EHS may subsequently be used to communicate findings and recommendations to patients and providers, with the ability to provide any subsequently required referrals. As patient's participate in LCS, tracking downstream appointments, procedures, and repeat imaging

studies becomes important and may pose a challenge. Certain EHSs may contain systems to allow for this, whereas other third-party software exists that at times can be integrated into the existing EHS.

As the use of the EHS continues to play a dynamic role in medical practice, there are also proposed future uses that may better identify patients who would benefit from LCS. A deep learning model was recently developed, and chest radiograph was used along with data extracted from the EHS to identify patients at high risk of lung cancer, including those not eligible by 2022 CMS criteria or where CMS eligibility was unknown.[31] A separate deep learning model has demonstrated accuracy in predicting lung cancer risk based on a single LDCT.[32] Continued model development and adaption may further expand LCS uptake and also expedite care by automated risk assessment.

INCORPORATION OF LUNG NODULE CLINIC

As results of LDCT are reported, the incorporation of a lung nodule clinic (LNC) can provide a mechanism for standardized follow-up when needed. In addition to managing screen-detected nodules, the LNC can also include an arm to capture incidental pulmonary nodules. Data demonstrate that more than 1.5 million incidental pulmonary nodules (IPNs) are identified annually. Cancer rates may actually be greater than those observed for LCS and are reported between 5% and 9%.[33,34] Follow-up can be challenging, especially as many IPNs are identified through imaging performed in the emergency department. Rates of guideline concordant follow-up are less than 40%, and underserved populations are at most risk.[35]

The complementary nature of LCS and IPN programs has been demonstrated, as both serve means to identify early-stage cancers.[36,37] A prospective observational study of patients cared for in the Mississippi Delta region, where poverty rates and socioeconomic distress levels are high, evaluated the utility of a lung nodule program to assist in the management of concerning lesions found outside of LCS. The nodule program in addition served as a safety net for patients with lung findings who would otherwise not be eligible for screening. Higher rates of stage I and II disease were found in both the LCS and IPN groups, as compared with those receiving standard multidisciplinary care. Curative intent surgery was also offered at higher rates in these groups, who subsequently enjoyed improved survival. Overall, IPN programs offer an alternative means to bridging the gap where LCS underestimates cancer risk, especially for women and patients of color.[36,38]

In addition, it is important to ensure a mechanism for the follow-up of other incidental findings.[16] LDCT may also identify pathology outside of the lung parenchyma, including concerning coronary calcification, lymphadenopathy, or breast lesions. Appropriate communication with patients and their primary care providers is essential, and programs must be prepared to manage this additional element of LDCT. The nurse navigators or other systems in place for LDCT result dissemination, including providers in the LNC, may similarly be used to convey and arrange follow-up of other concerning findings.

PUTTING THE PIECES TOGETHER: RESTRUCTURING A LUNG CANCER SCREENING PROGRAM AT AN URBAN ACADEMIC CENTER

The patients cared for within our health system encompass a diverse and heterogeneous group. In evaluating patients diagnosed with non–small cell lung cancer (NSCLC) at our institution between 2016 and 2019, 39% of patients were identified as Black, whereas 33% were Hispanic. Concerning among this population was the relative high proportion of patients diagnosed with metastatic disease compared with other hospitals in the country (45% vs 37%) and lower rates of stage I disease (25% vs 31%, **Fig. 1**). These numbers emphasized the need for earlier detection in our at-risk patient population. Investing in our LCS program,

especially given that smoking rates approach 14% in our community, became a priority in striving to improve outcomes associated with NSCLC.

Following the COVID-19 pandemic, the LCS program at our institution was largely underperforming. Resources had been reallocated to address needs of the pandemic leading to an understaffed program, which was coupled with decreased referrals and prolonged timing from referral to completion of LDCT. Following multidisciplinary discussion, LCS was transitioned from the Department of Radiology into a Cancer Center–administered collaborative effort led by thoracic surgery and radiology. Understanding the need for more resources to support functionality of the program, an additional nurse practitioner was allocated to provide screening navigation for patients. Cancer Center personnel were also organized into an access team to coordinate LDCT scheduling.

During this restructuring, the institution's cancer service line developed a 6-step approach to systematize the process of LCS and incorporate it within the institutional EHS (**Fig. 2**). First, a provider placed an order within the EHS to refer the patient for LCS. This referral is then routed to the access team within the Cancer Center who facilitates a telehealth visit with a dedicated nurse practitioner. During this visit, screening eligibility is confirmed, and patients participate in SDM to better understand the rationale, logistics, and process of LCS. With confirmed eligibility and patient agreement for screening, the NP then orders LDCT following which the access team obtains

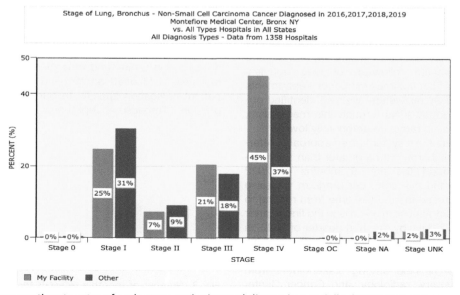

Fig. 1. Disproportionate rates of early stage and advanced disease in a racially diverse population.

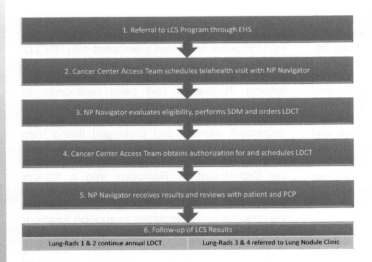

Fig. 2. Six steps of lung cancer screening at the Montefiore Einstein cancer center.

authorization for and schedules the study. After the scan is performed, the NP navigator receives the results and communicates this with the patient along with his or her primary care provider. In the last step, patients with Lung-Rads 1 and 2 results remained enrolled in LCS and are contacted annually by the NP navigator for continued screening, whereas Lung-Rads 3 and 4 patients are referred to our institutional lung nodule clinic for further discussion and management of findings.

The LNC was established toward the beginning of 2022 to assist management of both screen-detected and incidental pulmonary nodules. With the expansion of our screening program and corresponding identification of nodules requiring closer follow-up, the program identified the need for more formalized assessment of these patients. The LNC is staffed by members of thoracic surgery and interventional pulmonology. The primary objective of the LNC is to ensure appropriate and guideline-directed follow-up of lung nodules. With several high-volume emergency departments within our hospital system, we also identified potential to capture IPNs through this mechanism, where follow-up rates are notoriously low.[35]

As a result of this systematized approach, referrals climbed sharply with a greater than 150% increase through the first 9 months of 2022 (**Fig. 3**). During this time, our program was also able to decrease the median time from referral to LDCT appointment from 86 days in the first quarter of 2021 to 27 days by the third quarter of 2022. In order to maintain efficiency and afford scalability of the LCS program, monthly quality assurance meetings were held among stakeholders from thoracic surgery, radiology, and Cancer Center leadership. Monthly data along with issues related

to workflow, resource allocation, and outreach are discussed to maintain sustained growth. At the conclusion of 2022, our program has increased screening by 73% with 1628 completed scans compared with 943 the year prior.

DISCUSSION

The elements discussed earlier have each played an important role, as we have revamped our LCS program. Although we have encountered success with these processes in terms of increasing the number of patients completing LDCT, we acknowledge that further work is needed to capture the larger denominator of at-risk patients in our large, underserved community. To increase the uptake of and compliance with LCS, our institution has pursued further programmatic goals. Central to this initiative, project URBANA (Increasing Access to LUng Cancer ScReening in the Bronx in LAtinx and AfricaN American Communities) is focused on targeted education and patient navigation specific to our patient demographic. Through a 3-pronged approach, we

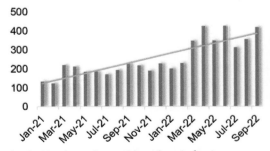

Fig. 3. Number of monthly referrals for lung cancer screening.

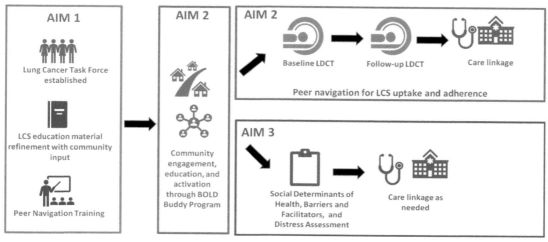

Fig. 4. Project URBANA implementation.

seek to improve access to LCS through a culturally sensitive educational program, institution of peer navigation to assist patients through the process, and better understanding of social determinants of health as a barrier to LCS (**Fig. 4**).

The importance of understanding the needs of the screening population has been previously stated. Accommodating this in practice requires outreach and collaboration with the community. To that end, we have incorporated a lung cancer task force where providers, lung cancer survivors, and community advocates come together to discuss barriers to screening. Educational materials will subsequently be tailored to incorporate cultural, language, and geographically specific needs with acceptability testing performed through the task force.

A more novel approach that will be included in this project is the use of trained peer navigators. Peer or lay navigators have demonstrated efficacy akin to professional patient navigators and can be cost-effective, sustainable social role models for patients who reinforce self-efficacy.[9] These programs are currently in use throughout our Cancer Center with favorable responses from patients. Expansion into LCS will include specific training from a diverse group of lung cancer survivors who will help elucidate the psychosocial and cultural barriers to LCS to facilitate uptake, treatment, and follow-up care. By conducting surveys of social determinants of health, our peer navigators may also generate further data to customize our screening approach.

As we continue to learn more about factors and techniques that may affect LCS rates, we additionally anticipate challenges that will require continuous adaptation of our program. Quality assurance meetings to review monthly data have identified 2 particular areas that our center has been working to address. As our referral volume has increased, we have had to maintain efficiency in ensuring scanner time and availability along with managing personnel to sustain the influx. With weekend and evening hours available to schedule LDCT, we have been able to maintain a short wait time from SDM to scan. An additional concern that has been raised is the high rate of nonattendance to scheduled LDCT appointments, which occurred in 36% of our patients in 2021. Although we have been able to increase and sustain referrals, this no-show rate comes at the cost of specifically allocated resources and time. Preliminary institutional data have revealed an association with first time screeners and current smokers and rates of no-show. We have therefore proposed an intervention focused on this cohort to improve adherence to scheduled LDCT.

Since the restructuring of our LCS program beginning in 2021, data collection has played an integral role in allowing our program to increase its reach throughout our community. We have also been enabled to apply for and receive competitive funding to carry out initiatives such as project URBANA and our IPN program. Although some of the metrics mentioned can contribute to the success of a centralized LCS program, individualization to local needs and ongoing adaptation are critical to the success of LCS.

SUMMARY

Clearly, developing a LCS program is a dynamic process that requires personnel and resources, organization, and time. Elements considered for incorporation include establishment of a multidisciplinary team that incorporates primary care input, assessment of the target population for potential barriers to care, effective utilization of the EHS, and incorporation of a lung nodule clinic. Perhaps most importantly, each screening program must be customized to accommodate practice patterns and the patient base in order to maximize uptake. As LCS completes a decade of evidence-based support and CMS approval, increasing participation must be a priority, as the identification and treatment of early-stage cancers should clearly increase overall survival from lung cancer.

CLINICS CARE POINTS

- LCS reduces mortality, and more efforts are required to expand screening to eligible patients.
- Different models of LCS exist, and each program should be individualized to the patients served.
- Several factors contribute to the successful development of a screening program and should be considered by all involved stakeholders to best overcome barriers to care.

FUNDING

NPC: 11/1/21-10/31-23 Lungevity Foundation, Chudgar PI; Investigating incidental pulmonary nodules in an underserved community. BMS: 10/18/21 – 9/30-23 Price Family Foundation Pilot Projects to Develop Experimental Cancer Therapeutics for Underrepresented Populations; Stiles, PI; Investigating the mechanistic relationship between ART1, a mono-ADP-ribosyltransferase, and the EGFR pathway in lung cancer 3/15/22 – 3/14/24 Bristol Myers Squibb Foundation; Stiles, Co-PI (Co-PIs: Alyson Moadel-Roblee, Lungevity Foundation); Project URBANA: Increasing access to lung cancer screening in the Bronx in Latinx and African American communities. 9/1/22 – 8/31/24 American Cancer Society; Stiles, Co-PI (Co-PI Vikas Mehta); Building Reliable Oncology Navigation, Centered Around Neoadjuvant Therapy: The BRONx-CAN project.

DISCLOSURE

N.P. Chudgar: none; B.M. Stiles: Medtronic, AstraZeneca, Genentech, Pfizer, Arcus Biosciences, Bristol Myers Squib, BMS Foundation, Gala Therapeutics, and the Lung Cancer Research Foundation.

REFERENCES

1. Aberle DR, Adams AM, Berg CD, et al. Reduced lung-cancer mortality with low-dose computed tomographic screening. N Engl J Med 2011; 365(5):395–409.
2. de Koning HJ, van der Aalst CM, de Jong PA, et al. Reduced Lung-Cancer Mortality with Volume CT Screening in a Randomized Trial. N Engl J Med 2020;382(6):503–13.
3. Pastorino U, Silva M, Sestini S, et al. Prolonged lung cancer screening reduced 10-year mortality in the MILD trial: new confirmation of lung cancer screening efficacy. Ann Oncol 2019;30(7):1162–9 [published correction appears in Ann Oncol. 2019 Oct 1;30(10):1672].
4. Jemal A, Fedewa SA. Lung Cancer Screening With Low-Dose Computed Tomography in the United States-2010 to 2015. JAMA Oncol 2017;3(9): 1278–81.
5. Lake M, Shusted CS, Juon HS, et al. Black patients referred to a lung cancer screening program experience lower rates of screening and longer time to follow-up. BMC Cancer 2020;20(1):561.
6. Watson L, Cotter MM, Shafer S, et al. Implementation of a Lung Cancer Screening Program in Two Federally Qualified Health Centers. Public Health Rep 2021;136(4):397–402.
7. Merzel CR, Isasi CR, Strizich G, et al. Smoking cessation among U.S. Hispanic/Latino adults: Findings from the Hispanic Community Health Study/Study of Latinos (HCHS/SOL). Prev Med 2015;81: 412–9.
8. Quaife SL, Marlow LAV, McEwen A, et al. Attitudes towards lung cancer screening in socioeconomically deprived and heavy smoking communities: informing screening communication. Health Expect 2017; 20(4):563–73.
9. Lopez-Olivo MA, Maki KG, Choi NJ, et al. Patient Adherence to Screening for Lung Cancer in the US: A Systematic Review and Meta-analysis. JAMA Netw Open 2020;3:e2025102.
10. Batile JC, Maroules CD, Latif MA, et al. A five-step strategy for building an LDCT lung cancer screening program. Appl Radiol 2018;47(1):12–8.
11. Sakoda LC, Rivera MP, Zhang J, et al. Patterns and Factors Associated With Adherence to Lung Cancer Screening in Diverse Practice Settings. JAMA Netw Open 2021;4(4):e218559.
12. Smith HB, Ward R, Frazier C, et al. Guideline-Recommended Lung Cancer Screening Adherence Is Superior With a Centralized Approach. Chest 2022; 161(3):818–25.

13. Núñez ER, Triplette M. Addressing Lung Cancer Screening Disparities: What Does It Mean to Be Centralized? Ann Am Thorac Soc 2022;19(9):1457–8.

14. Bernstein MA, Ronk M, Ebright MI. Establishing a lung cancer screening program in a non-university hospital. AME Med J 2018;3:102.

15. Lewis JA, Chen H, Weaver KE, et al. Low Provider Knowledge Is Associated With Less Evidence-Based Lung Cancer Screening. J Natl Compr Canc Netw 2019;17(4):339–46.

16. Sands J, Tammemägi MC, Couraud S, et al. Lung Screening Benefits and Challenges: A Review of The Data and Outline for Implementation. J Thorac Oncol 2021;16(1):37–53.

17. Allen CG, Cotter MM, Smith RA, et al. Successes and challenges of implementing a lung cancer screening program in federally qualified health centers: a qualitative analysis using the Consolidated Framework for Implementation Research. Transl Behav Med 2021;11(5):1088–98.

18. Fintelmann FJ, Bernheim A, Digumarthy SR, et al. The 10 Pillars of Lung Cancer Screening: Rationale and Logistics of a Lung Cancer Screening Program. Radiographics 2015;35(7):1893–908.

19. McKee BJ, McKee AB, Kitts AB, et al. Low-dose computed tomography screening for lung cancer in a clinical setting: essential elements of a screening program. J Thorac Imaging 2015;30(2):115–29.

20. Doerfler-Evans RE. Shifting paradigms continued-the emergence and the role of nurse navigator. J Thorac Dis 2016;8(Suppl 6):S498–500.

21. Watson J, Broome ME, Schneider SM. Low-Dose Computed Tomography: Effects of Oncology Nurse Navigation on Lung Cancer Screening. Clin J Oncol Nurs 2020;24(4):421–9.

22. Randhawa S, Moore RF, DiSesa V, et al. Role of Thoracic Surgeons in Lung Cancer Screening: Opportune Time for Involvement. J Thorac Oncol 2018;13(3):298–300.

23. Stiles BM, Pua B, Altorki NK. Screening for Lung Cancer. Surg Oncol Clin N Am 2016;25(3):469–79.

24. Ho H, Williamson C, Regis SM, et al. Surgery and invasive diagnostic procedures for benign disease are rare in a large low-dose computed tomography lung cancer screening program. J Thorac Cardiovasc Surg 2021;161(3):790–802.

25. Fedewa SA, Kazerooni EA, Studts JL, et al. State Variation in Low-Dose Computed Tomography Scanning for Lung Cancer Screening in the United States. J Natl Cancer Inst 2021;113(8):1044–52.

26. Su CT, Bhargava A, Shah CD, et al. Screening Patterns and Mortality Differences in Patients With Lung Cancer at an Urban Underserved Community. Clin Lung Cancer 2018;19(5):e767–73.

27. DuBard CA, Gizlice Z. Language spoken and differences in health status, access to care, and receipt of preventive services among US Hispanics. Am J Public Health 2008;98(11):2021–8.

28. Haddad DN, Sandler KL, Henderson LM, et al. Disparities in Lung Cancer Screening: A Review. Ann Am Thorac Soc 2020;17(4):399–405.

29. Fathi JT, White CS, Greenberg GM, et al. The Integral Role of the Electronic Health Record and Tracking Software in the Implementation of Lung Cancer Screening-A Call to Action to Developers: A White Paper From the National Lung Cancer Roundtable. Chest 2020;157(6):1674–9.

30. Modin HE, Fathi JT, Gilbert CR, et al. Pack-Year Cigarette Smoking History for Determination of Lung Cancer Screening Eligibility. Comparison of the Electronic Medical Record versus a Shared Decision-making Conversation. Ann Am Thorac Soc 2017;14(8):1320–5.

31. Raghu VK, Walia AS, Zinzuwadia AN, et al. Validation of a Deep Learning-Based Model to Predict Lung Cancer Risk Using Chest Radiographs and Electronic Medical Record Data. JAMA Netw Open 2022;5(12):e2248793.

32. Mikhael PG, Wohlwend J, Yala A, et al. Sybil: A Validated Deep Learning Model to Predict Future Lung Cancer Risk From a Single Low-Dose Chest Computed Tomography. J Clin Oncol 2023;41(12):2191–200.

33. Gould MK, Tang T, Liu IL, et al. Recent Trends in the Identification of Incidental Pulmonary Nodules. Am J Respir Crit Care Med 2015;192(10):1208–14.

34. Wiener RS, Gould MK, Slatore CG, et al. Resource use and guideline concordance in evaluation of pulmonary nodules for cancer: too much and too little care. JAMA Intern Med 2014;174(6):871–80.

35. Farjah F, Monsell SE, Gould MK, et al. Association of the Intensity of Diagnostic Evaluation With Outcomes in Incidentally Detected Lung Nodules. JAMA Intern Med 2021;181(4):480–9.

36. Osarogiagbon RU, Liao W, Faris NR, et al. Lung Cancer Diagnosed Through Screening, Lung Nodule, and Neither Program: A Prospective Observational Study of the Detecting Early Lung Cancer (DELUGE) in the Mississippi Delta Cohort. J Clin Oncol 2022;40(19):2094–105.

37. LeMense GP, Waller EA, Campbell C, et al. Development and outcomes of a comprehensive multidisciplinary incidental lung nodule and lung cancer screening program. BMC Pulm Med 2020;20(1):115.

38. Pinsky PF, Lau YK, Doubeni CA. Potential Disparities by Sex and Race or Ethnicity in Lung Cancer Screening Eligibility Rates. Chest 2021;160(1):341–50.

Barriers to Lung Cancer Screening Access from the Perspective of the Patient and Current Interventions

Katherine T. Leopold, BS[a], Lisa Carter-Bawa, PhD, MPH, APRN, ANP-C, FAAN[b],*

KEYWORDS

- Lung cancer screening • Cancer screening • Barriers • Access • Patient barriers

KEY POINTS

- Patient barriers to lung cancer screening (LCS) include cognitive factors (lack of awareness, limited information/misinformation, and low perceived risk), factors related to access (logistical issues, lack of provider recommendation, cost, and other financial/social factors), and psychological factors (fear, fatalism, lung cancer worry, and stigma).
- Current interventions aim to address patient barriers and have had varying degrees of success with most research focusing on cognitive factors and factors related to access.
- More research is needed to determine which interventions best address patient barriers to LCS.

INTRODUCTION

Lung cancer is the leading cause of cancer-related deaths in the United States causing an estimated 350 deaths per day.[1] Lung cancer outcomes largely depend on early diagnosis; distant-stage disease has an abysmal 6% 5-year relative survival rate as compared with 33% for regional stage and 60% for localized disease.[1] Low-dose computed tomography (LDCT) of the chest is the gold standard for lung cancer screening (LCS). The US Preventive Services Task Force (USPSTF) issued an official recommendation in 2013 for LCS with LDCT of the chest largely based on the National Lung Screening Trial—the largest randomized controlled trial to date—which showed a 20% reduction in mortality among participants who received chest LDCT screening as compared with chest x-ray.[2,3] In addition, scientific evidence from prior studies in the late 1990s and 2000s confirmed the efficacy and mortality reduction associated with chest LDCT.[3,4]

Although lung screening is recommended by the USPSTF, has the potential to detect lung cancer at earlier, more treatable stages, has a 20% lung cancer-related mortality reduction in individuals at risk and is covered by Medicare and other health insurers, population uptake has been challenging.[3] It has been a decade since the USPSTF released its recommendation, yet less than 6% of screening-eligible Americans have been screened.[5] Screening-eligible individuals are generally unaware of early detection of lung cancer. Our team's prior work revealed that in addition to lack of awareness, screening-eligible individuals in the United States do not screen—*when they are aware*—because of perceived barriers to screening.[6–10] Because researchers have explored implementation and dissemination efforts of this relatively new screening option, research examining patient barriers and facilitators to LCS have been fairly well characterized in many populations in the United States. Researchers

[a] Hackensack University School of Medicine, 123 Metro Boulevard, Nutley, NJ 07110, USA; [b] Cancer Prevention Precision Control Institute, Center for Discovery & Innovation, at Hackensack Meridian Health, 111 Ideation Way, B430, Nutley, NJ 07110, USA
* Corresponding author. Center for Discovery & Innovation, Cancer Prevention Precision Control Institute, 111 Ideation Way, Nutley, NJ 07110.
E-mail address: Lisa.CarterBawa@hmh-cdi.org

Thorac Surg Clin 33 (2023) 343–351
https://doi.org/10.1016/j.thorsurg.2023.04.003
1547-4127/23/© 2023 Elsevier Inc. All rights reserved.

now have the opportunity to begin exploring interventions that address these barriers. This article discusses patient barriers to LCS in the United States and proposed interventions to date (**Fig. 1**).

CONCEPTUAL FRAMEWORK

As we consider barriers to LCS, we can contextualize them within the larger multilevel framework from the patient perspective of the Conceptual Model for Lung Cancer Screening Participation which notes shared decision-making (SDM) as critical in the context of lung cancer screening (LCS).[11] The SDM process between the patient and clinician is a dyadic interaction that is influenced by multiple variables as a patient progresses through the health-care system. However, this introduces the potential for barriers to accessing LCS at different touch points within the health-care system. Patient barriers to LCS can be characterized as psychological factors, cognitive factors, and factors related to use. The following will discuss these categories.

BARRIERS TO LUNG CANCER SCREENING: COGNITIVE FACTORS

Cognitive factors such as lack of awareness, limited information/misinformation, and low perceived risk of lung cancer act as patient barriers to LCS.[6,9,12] As LCS is relatively new, many patients are not familiar with the national screening guideline.[4,12] A lack of awareness among providers could further compound lack of patient awareness by creating missed opportunities for eligible patients to learn about and complete screening.[6,12] Among eligible patients who are aware that LCS exists, the novelty of the scan may also contribute to the barrier to screening secondary to misunderstanding.[6,12] Patients may not realize that they are eligible for screening or

may not understand the potential benefits of screening for them personally.[6,12] Patients with low perceived risk of lung cancer and those who feel healthy may find screening unnecessary.[12]

Most interventions designed to address barriers have focused on cognitive factors. Researchers have explored increasing awareness and understanding of LCS using educational materials and community-based health education. Educational materials include strategies such as leaflet distribution, film and television media, social media, and decision aids.

The National Health Service (NHS) in the United Kingdom has developed and refined educational leaflets on LCS to potentially eligible citizens. Quaife and colleagues (2020) observed that having a low burden, stepped leaflet focused on patient barriers was not a critical factor in achieving improved screening but that leaflet distribution had a positive outcome on screening participation during the Lung Screening Uptake Trial (LSUT).[13] LCS uptake in LSUT was 52.6% with no significant difference in uptake between the control (52.9%) and intervention (52.3%) groups (OR, 0.98; 95% CI, 0.82–1.170).[13] Jallow and colleagues (2022) in an NHS-funded in England entitled "Targeted Lung Health Check" showed that individuals find leaflets acceptable but alone they may not be enough to guide a patient through an SDM model.[14] Together, the studies indicate the benefit of a physical reminder/promoter of LCS where the target population and message may be optimized for greatest effect.

Use of video-based educational strategies such as films led to a similar dichotomy in outcomes. Ruperal and colleagues (2019) showed that participants in LSUT who received both an informational film and a booklet had a larger improvement in knowledge (β coefficient 0.32; CI, 0.05–0.58; $P = .02$) compared with the participants who received only a booklet but that the strategy did not ultimately affect uptake.[15] The Terminate Lung Cancer study in Kentucky initially intended to use television advertisements to increase LCS awareness but was unable to carry them out due to cost limitations.[16] Although television may prove an effective strategy to increase awareness, costs may prevent such a strategy from being implemented on a wide scale.

Strategies involving information dissemination through social media bear a similarity to video-based strategies such as film or television. Jessup and colleagues (2018) used pay-per-click advertisements on social media linking patients, providers, and caregivers to educational content. This approach increased visits to institutional educational webpages and prompted participants

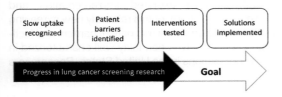

Fig. 1. Progress in LCS research. Once slow uptake of low-dose computerized tomography (LDCT) for LCS was recognized, investigators began to identify patient barriers to LCS. Recent research has focused on testing interventions to address these patient barriers. This article summarizes current interventions and highlights opportunities for future interventions that, when implemented, will overcome patient barriers.

to schedule LDCT examinations.[17] The campaign encouraged a marginal increase in mean scheduled LDCT per week of 3% during and 5.8% 1-week postcampaign ($P = .001$).[17]

Decision aids prompt interactive participation by participants and personalize the educational strategy, potentially drawing subjects into the process of opting for screening. Decision aids must be delivered through a written, video, face-to-face, or virtual medium, and investigators have reported success using a variety of strategies. Lillie and colleagues (2017) reported that decision tools influence Veterans' perceptions about LCS decision-making factors.[18] Exposure to Direct LCS Invitation (with an associated decision aid) increased Veterans' attention to specific decision-making factors (benefits, harms, and neutral factors).[18] Housten and colleagues (2018) used a video-based patient LCS decision aid and increased knowledge by 33% posttest (M = 3.97, SD = 2.87, 95% CI 2.90–5.04, $P < .001$).[19] Lau and colleagues (2015) used a web-based decision aid and showed that knowledge of risk factors, benign lumps, and screening benefits, harms, and eligibility factors increased (pretest M = 7.52/14, SD = 1.89; posttest M = 10.93/14, SD = 2.19, $P < .001$) and that decisional conflict decreased (pretest M = 46.33, SD = 29.69; posttest M = 15.08, SD = 25.78, $P < .001$).[20] Finally, Mazzone and colleagues (2017) combined face-to-face counseling with video, and web-based decision aids leading to increased knowledge of LCS eligibility for age ($P < .0001$), smoking history ($P < .0001$), benefits ($P = .03$), and harms ($P \leq .0001$).[21] Of 423 participants who had an SDM visit, only 23 (5.4%) did not go on to have LDCT.[21] Considered together, the data on use of decision aids suggest broad success when delivered in a variety of platforms.

Education can also take place in a group or community setting. Community-based mechanisms typically depend on members of the target population as organizers and/or instructors to help participants gain a level of comfort and trust with the people who are delivering the information. Leng and colleagues (2022), for example, reported that Chinese livery drivers in NYC found the idea of community health workers (CHWs) acceptable as a potential intervention to increase LCS.[22] Although CHWs may open a line of communication with target populations, the ultimate success of community-based programs will likely depend on achieving the same level of interaction that has been observed using SDM as described above and identifying a good match between messengers and the target population. Bouchard and colleagues (2022) had CHWs led community health

education sessions on LCS in a variety of different formats, hosting both individual and group sessions and sessions in-person, virtually, and over the phone.[23] In all formats, Bouchard and colleagues (2022) discovered that LCS knowledge increased but that one-on-one phone calls were most effective at reaching participants who were older, had lower incomes, more current smoking, smoked for more years, more cigarettes per day, lower preintervention LCS knowledge, and higher preintervention fear and worry.[23] Williams and colleagues (2021) found a productive formula pairing CHWs with a population of black women to increase participant knowledge of LCS.[24] CHWs were trained to deliver 4 90-minute sessions addressing the core constructs of the Health Beliefs Model in relation to LCS to participants at community sites (churches, federally qualified health centers [FQHCs], and recreation center) during the course of 4 weeks.[24] Using this strategy from 2015 to 2017, Williams and colleagues (2021) achieved a knowledge increase regarding LCS ($P = .001$), decreases in both perceived severity and perceived barriers ($P = .001$), as well as an increase in positive responses to perceived benefits of LCS. Importantly, more than one-third of eligible participants chose to participate in LDCT screening and more than half of tobacco-using participants engaged in a cessation program.[24]

Not all reports of community-based strategies have proved as feasible. Kathuria and colleagues (2022) focused on an inpatient population to evaluate SDM with a nurse practitioner paired with CHWs to assess improvements in uptake of LCS.[25] The fact that many inpatients had already received diagnostic CTs and were ineligible for screening resulted in a limited study population in which 50% (5/10) of participants in the Inpatient SDM + CHW-navigation group completed LCS, whereas 9% (1/11) in the comparator group, dissemination of a decision aid and encouragement to follow up with primary care provider (PCP), completed LCS ($P < .05$).[25] This approach deserves evaluation in a larger population, perhaps in an outpatient setting.[25]

Physician-led educational sessions in the community may be effective at increasing participant understanding of LCS. Sakoda and colleagues (2020) reported that educational classes focused on LCS and taught by physician specialists (usually pulmonologists) increased knowledge among participants by 51% posttest (M = 0.09, SD = 2.29, $P < .0001$).[26] Fung and colleagues (2018) described a randomized control trial exploring the efficacy of cancer prevention seminars, conducted by culturally and linguistically competent physicians and a health education team.[27] When compared the outcomes in the control group (a series of seminars focused on biospecimen education), participants in the LCS seminars had statistically insignificant increased awareness of the importance of early detection of lung cancer.[27]

BARRIERS TO LUNG CANCER SCREENING: FACTORS RELATED TO ACCESS

Factors impeding access to LCS include logistical issues, lack of clinician recommendation, cost, and other financial/social barriers.[6,12] Access to LCS varies internationally depending on each country's health-care system structure and screening guidelines. Most public and private health insurance plans cover LCS in the United States; however, not all people living in the United States are eligible for or can afford health insurance.[28] Screenings covered by health insurance may incur indirect costs such as travel expenses and time off work. For patients who screen positive, downstream testing may not be covered by health insurance.[6] The process of scheduling a screening may also prove daunting for patients busy with financial or social concerns. Long traveling distance to screening, limited hours of operation, and insufficient support staff for LCS programming could also affect a patient's ability to schedule and attend LCS.[6,12]

Interventions addressing factors related to access to LCS range from direct outreach to structural change. Direct outreach efforts include targeted telephone outreach and use of patient navigators to connect patients to screening. The Yorkshire Lung Screening Trial (YLST) using mail invitation and telephone triage for responders to assess LCS eligibility before referral to local mobile screening units.[29] A total of 22,815 individuals (50.8%) responded to the mailed invitations, of which 6650 eventually received LCS after the YLST team confirmed eligibility.[29] Patients who were currently smoking (adjusted OR 0.73, 95% CI 0.62–0.87) and were socioeconomically deprived (adjusted OR 0.78, 95% CI 0.62–0.98) had lower LCS uptake.[29] Dickson and colleagues (2022) found that telephone risk assessment increased the proportion of in-person LCS eligibility assessment attendees eligible for screening (60.3% without phone screening vs 82.6% with phone screening, $P < .001$) but congruence between phone and in-person eligibility assessment was lower in younger patients and minority groups.[30] Telephone risk assessment addresses the barrier of travel to appointments by remotely confirming eligibility for LCS, yet it does not address factors that make patients less likely to

call initially such as limited time or access to telephone service among the poor.

Patient navigation improves cancer screening uptake in populations with barriers related to access. Patient navigators are linguistically, culturally, competent health professionals trained to connect underserved patients to the health-care system. Perac-Lima and colleagues (2018) explored the use of patient navigators to increase LCS uptake among current smokers who were patients at community health centers associated with Massachusetts General Hospital.[31] Patient navigators called eligible patients directly to discuss risks/benefits of screening, their barriers to LCS, strategies to overcome those barriers, and the importance of discussing LCS with their PCP.[31] Then, patient navigators arranged appointments for interested patients to complete SDM with their PCP. Compared with patients who received usual care (PCP invitation), patients who received the intervention (PCP invitation plus patient navigator services) were more likely to receive any chest CT (31.0% [124] vs 17.3% [138], $P < .001$) and LDCT specifically for LCS (23.5% [94] vs 8.6% [69], $P < .001$).[31] CHWs, mentioned above in the "Barriers to lung cancer screening: cognitive factors" section, may also conduct patient navigation to LCS in addition to their role as community educators.

Beyond direct outreach, researchers have considered adjusting the structure of the health-care system to better accommodate patient access barriers to LCS using mobile CT scanners, free screenings, and staff dedicated to improving LCS uptake. Crosbie and colleagues (2019) parked mobile CT screening vans outside of shopping centers in Manchester, United Kingdom, and conducted eligibility assessments and LCS for high-risk participants on the spot.[32] Most participants were ranked in the United Kingdom's lowest deprivation quintile (75% or n = 1893/2541), more than half were high-risk for lung cancer (56% or 1423/2541), and more than half completed LCS (55% or 1384/2541); of those screened, 3% (95% CI 2.3% to 4.1%) were diagnosed with lung cancer.[32] Chiarantano and colleagues (2022) used both mobile CT units and primary health-care offices to recruit high-risk participants for a lung cancer and screening program in Brazil.[33] All participants (n = 233) were offered smoking cessation counseling and received LCS, and 3 participants (1.3%) were diagnosed with lung cancer.[33] Chiarantano and colleagues (2022) report that recruitment proved a challenge for the program, yet more than half (55.8%) of the program's participants were recruited in just 2 days of mobile health unit use.[33] Bartlett and colleagues (2020) in

London, United Kingdom, directly compared participant response to invitation to screen at local mobile versus hospital-based CT scanners. Bartlett and colleagues (2022) found no significant difference in participant response to each site (20.4% 1047/5135 responded to hospital site invitation, 21.7% 702/3231 responded to mobile site invitation, $P = .14$) with significantly shorter travel distance for patients traveling to a hospital site versus mobile site (3.3 vs 6.4 km, $P < .01$) suggesting that both location types regardless of travel distance are effective.[34] Incorporation of mobile CT units is a feasible structural change, which may be targeted toward underserved areas; however, it is unclear whether mobile CT units are significantly more accessible than hospital-based screening.

On a system level, cost and staff support influence access to LCS. Hochheimer and colleagues (2021) examined factors influencing LCS uptake between 2012 and 2016 at 3 types of primary care practices across 8 states: urban safety net practices with high proportions of uninsured and Black patients, suburban private practices serving an affluent, educated population, and FQHCs in rural, suburban, urban, and academic settings.[35] Among these 3 clusters, only the urban safety net practices significantly increased LCS uptake, nearly doubling their baseline screening rate (10.4%–19.1%, $P < .01$).[35] Hochheimer and colleagues (2021) attributed the success of urban safety net practices to full time staff to promote their LCS program and free LCS regardless of health insurance status.[35] Explicitly promoting LCS through full-time staff focused on lung cancer prevention increased LCS more than relying solely on clinician referral to LCS.

BARRIERS TO LUNG CANCER SCREENING: PSYCHOLOGICAL FACTORS

Psychosocial factors such as fear, fatalism, lung cancer worry, medical mistrust, and perceived stigma have the potential to serve as a critical barrier to LCS.[6,8,10,12] Individuals eligible for LCS have a history of smoking long-term and may perceive their risk of lung cancer higher secondary to their heavy smoking history.[10] In some people, this may evoke a fear of being diagnosed with lung cancer because of the perceived higher risk.[6,10,12] Research in breast cancer screening has demonstrated that a small-to-moderate amount of fear can actually influence someone to be screened.[36] However, they found that high levels of fear served as a barrier to screening because the individual could not make the decision to move forward with screening because of

their fear.[36] Fear and fatalism are closely related. Lung cancer fatalism is defined as the belief that being diagnosed with lung cancer will result in death.[10] Fatalism has been shown to be a barrier to eligible individuals being screened for lung cancer. Some individuals who have smoked long-term and perceive their risk for lung cancer to be high may also think that there is nothing that can be done attributing a divine will to their potential diagnosis of lung cancer.[10] In this situation, these individuals do not necessarily see the value in screening for lung cancer because they view the situation as static. Lung cancer worry is an emotional reaction to the threat of lung cancer.[10] Moderate levels of cancer worry have been associated with delaying screening mammography in high-risk women.[37] Similarly, cancer worry about the results of cervical cancer screening was also identified as an important psychosocial barrier to the screening process.[38]

Perceived smoking-related stigma has been described by screening-eligible individuals as a key barrier to LCS as well as noted to be negatively associated with medical help-seeking behavior in individuals with symptoms suggestive of lung cancer.[10] Patients diagnosed with lung cancer fear shame and blame for the disease because of perceptions that family and friends will think the lung cancer was self-inflicted by smoking. Historically, perceptions of stigma have the potential to be a powerful barrier to cancer screening. Similarly, medical mistrust has been identified as a powerful barrier to LCS among eligible individuals. People have described mistrust of the health care system, mistrust of the government, and mistrust of the tobacco industry while noting uncertainty that LCS has any.[6,10,12] Medical mistrust has also been positively associated with late-stage lung cancer presentation primarily among ethnic minorities and vulnerable patient populations.[39] Medical mistrust is the belief that the health-care system itself and those working within it are untrustworthy, which has the potential to cascade into an impedance to LCS participation overall.

As of yet, few interventions have been used to address the psychological factors preventing patients from completing LCS. Quaife and colleagues (2020) created a leaflet specifically targeting psychological barriers (fear, fatalism, and stigma) to be disseminated using a low burden, stepped strategy during the LSUT.[13] LCS uptake was not significantly different among participants who received the leaflet targeting psychological barriers compared with those who received a standard information booklet.[13] Targeting psychological barriers may be sufficiently complex that a personalized approach, more active

Table 1
Barriers to, interventions for, and lessons learned about lung cancer screening

Barrier Type	Barriers	Past Interventions	Lessons Learned from Past Interventions
Cognitive factors	• Lack of awareness • Limited information/misinformation • Low perceived risk	• Leaflet distribution • Film and television media • Social media • Decision aids • CHWs • Community-based health education sessions	• Leaflet distribution is a cost-effective strategy to increase awareness for large populations • Film/television media, social media are engaging strategies to increase awareness • Decision aids can increase understanding of LCS, especially when combined with engaging dissemination strategies (film, social media) and face-to-face counseling • Culturally, linguistically competent education from CHWs and clinicians can increase awareness and understanding of LCS
Factors related to access	• Logistical issues • Lack of provider recommendation • Cost • Other financial/social factors	• Targeted telephone outreach • Patient navigation • Mobile CT scanners • Free screenings • Dedicated staff	• Targeted telephone outreach is acceptable, effective, further exploration needed to ensure equitable access for all populations • Patient navigation can address personal patient access barriers • Mobile CT scanners are as effective as fixed screening sites • Health systems that implement free screenings and having dedicated staff promoting screenings can increase uptake
Psychological factors	• Fear • Fatalism • Lung cancer worry • Medical mistrust • Stigma	• Educational material focused on psychological barriers • Community-based health education sessions adapted to include stigma	• Leaflets alone increase awareness of LCS but may need further supplementation to address psychological barriers • Adapting effective educational interventions to including information about psychological barriers may be effective

engagement with participants, or a larger system wide intervention may be required.[13]

Williams' initial study, referenced above in "Barriers to lung cancer screening: cognitive factors" section, was promising in terms of reducing cognitive barriers but no significant changes were observed in some psychological measures such as perceived susceptibility, perceived threat, or intent.[24] After completing the initial study between 2015 and 2017, Williams and colleagues (2021) conducted educational sessions from 2018 to 2019 with CHWs in a new area using curriculum updated to address lung cancer stigma.[40] Williams and colleagues (2021) repeated the success of the initial study with significant increases in lung cancer knowledge ($P \leq .0001$) and in perceived benefits of screening ($P = .034$); notably, the updated curriculum yielded decreases in lung cancer stigma ($P = .024$).[40] The success of Williams and colleagues (2021) in decreasing lung cancer stigma through education suggests that increased knowledge and understanding of LCS paired with education about lung cancer stigma could address barriers that are psychological factors in addition to barriers that are cognitive factors.[40]

DISCUSSION
Summary

LDCT of the chest is the gold standard for LCS. Even with this knowledge, many at-risk patients do not take advantage of this relatively simple, noninvasive screening procedure. A number of studies have identified barriers to screening with most generally classified as cognitive barriers, access barriers, and psychological barriers (**Table 1**). The state of the science has advanced from descriptive studies to understand LCS behavior toward intervention development and a key component of current interventions is to mitigate barriers (see **Table 1**). Interventions aimed at overcoming cognitive barriers have included educational materials, community-based leaflet distribution, film and television media campaigns, social media campaigns, and decision aids to support the patient–clinician discussion about LCS.[13–21] Another strategy has been to engage CHWs and other clinicians in educational efforts that target individuals eligible for screening, use of decision aids, and use of social media to increase awareness.[12–27] Similarly, evidence-based strategies to overcome cognitive barriers to screening include the use of CHWs as well as decision aids, particularly the practice of pairing the decision aid with face-to-face counseling or presented in a video format.[18–21] Use of CHWs has also been shown effective, especially where they are members of the community or have cultural competence.[23–25] To overcome access barriers, investigators have used targeted telephone outreach, patient navigation, mobile CT scanners, free screenings, and staff dedicated to LCS promotion. Having staff dedicated to both patient navigation and program coordination had a significant impact on LCS uptake.[29–35] Targeted telephone outreach effectively increased LCS uptake but needs further exploration to ensure that all populations have equitable access to screening.[29,30] Mobile CT scanners demonstrate effectiveness in areas not otherwise served by medical facilities.[32,33] Finally, the issue of psychological barriers to screening has received little attention. Most notably, to date, there is only one intervention that effectively positively influenced psychological barriers to screening (Williams and

colleagues 2022); this intervention was adapted to include CHW-led educational sessions regarding stigma once proven effective at addressing cognitive barriers to screening (ie, limited understanding of lung cancer and LCS).[40] Other interventions that successfully address cognitive factors such as decision aids could also be adapted to include information about psychological barriers in the future.

Future Directions

Although access to LCS is influenced by many factors at multiple levels, in order to address cancer health disparities, it is critical to continue to identify populations that are potentially vulnerable for inequities in access. As the science continues to advance, it is important that research to develop and implement evidence-based interventions that target specific factors to mitigate barriers to access be designed to foster engagement from the varied populations eligible for LCS. In addition, it is critical to design evidence-based interventions that are culturally competent, consider the varied ways people like to learn, and mitigate any potential for stigma by using person-first language and avoiding stigmatizing messaging. Future research is also needed that examines the combination of evidence-based strategies to determine if a particular combination provides a synergistic effect at mitigating access barriers. This may be accomplished by using novel study designs such as a multiphase optimization strategy or sequential multiple assignment randomized trial and should be considered.

CLINICS CARE POINTS

- Continue developing evidence-based interventions that have proven effective at addressing cognitive barriers, barriers to access, and psychological barriers.
- Adapt known effective interventions to different populations based on their cultural, linguistic needs.
- Enhance the focus on identifying interventions that could address psychological barriers to LCS.
- Encourage health systems to integrate evidence-based interventions into the standard care process.

DISCLOSURE

The authors have nothing to disclose.

REFERENCES

1. Siegel RL, Miller KD, Fuchs HE, et al. Cancer statistics, 2022. CA Cancer J Clin 2022. https://doi.org/10.3322/caac.21708.
2. Moyer VA, U.S. Preventive Services Task Force. Screening for lung cancer: U.S. Preventive Services Task Force recommendation statement. Ann Intern Med 2014;160(5):330–8.
3. Aberle DR, Adams AM, Berg CD, et al, National Lung Screening Trial Research Team. Reduced lung-cancer mortality with low-dose computed tomographic screening. N Engl J Med 2011;365(5):395–409.
4. Sharma D, Newman TG, Aronow WS. Lung cancer screening: history, current perspectives, and future directions. Arch Med Sci 2015;11(5):1033–43.
5. State of Lung Cancer. American Lung Association. 2022. Available at: https://www.lung.org/research/state-of-lung-cancer. Accessed May 5, 2023.
6. Carter-Harris L, Gould MK. Multilevel Barriers to the Successful Implementation of Lung Cancer Screening: Why Does It Have to Be So Hard? Ann Am Thorac Soc 2017;14(8):1261–5.
7. Carter-Harris L, Ceppa DP, Hanna N, et al. Lung cancer screening: what do long-term smokers know and believe? Health Expect 2017;20(1):59–68.
8. Carter-Harris L, Brandzel S, Wernli KJ, et al. A qualitative study exploring why individuals opt out of lung cancer screening. Fam Pract 2017;34(2):239–44.
9. Carter-Harris L, Slaven JE 2nd, Monahan PO, et al. Understanding lung cancer screening behaviour using path analysis. J Med Screen 2020;27(2):105–12 [published correction appears in J Med Screen. 2019 Nov 5;:969141319888037].
10. Carter-Harris L. Hidden in plain sight: psychological barriers to participation in lung cancer screening. Thorax 2020;75(12):1033–4.
11. Carter-Harris L, Davis LL, Rawl SM. Lung Cancer Screening Participation: Developing a Conceptual Model to Guide Research. Res Theor Nurs Pract 2016;30(4):333–52.
12. Cavers D, Nelson M, Rostron J, et al. Understanding patient barriers and facilitators to uptake of lung screening using low dose computed tomography: a mixed methods scoping review of the current literature. Respir Res 2022;23(1):374.
13. Quaife SL, Ruparel M, Dickson JL, et al. Lung screen uptake trial (LSUT): randomized controlled clinical trial testing targeted invitation materials. Am J Respir Crit Care Med 2020;201(8):965–75.
14. Jallow M, Black G, van Os S, et al. Acceptability of a standalone written leaflet for the National Health Service for England Targeted Lung Health Check Programme: A concurrent, think-aloud study. Health Expect 2022;25(4):1776–88.
15. Ruparel M, Quaife SL, Ghimire B, et al. Impact of a lung cancer screening information film on informed decision-making: a randomized trial. Ann Am Thorac Soc 2019;16(6):744–51.
16. Cardarelli R, Reese D, Roper KL, et al. Terminate lung cancer (TLC) study-A mixed-methods population approach to increase lung cancer screening awareness and low-dose computed tomography in Eastern Kentucky. Cancer Epidemiol 2017;46:1–8.
17. Jessup DL, Glover Iv M, Daye D, et al. Implementation of digital awareness strategies to engage patients and providers in a lung cancer screening program: retrospective study. J Med Internet Res 2018;20(2):e52.
18. Lillie SE, Fu SS, Fabbrini AE, et al. What factors do patients consider most important in making lung cancer screening decisions? Findings from a demonstration project conducted in the Veterans Health Administration. Lung Cancer 2017;104:38–44.
19. Housten AJ, Lowenstein LM, Leal VB, et al. Responsiveness of a brief measure of lung cancer screening knowledge. J Cancer Educ 2018;33(4):842–6.
20. Lau YK, Caverly TJ, Cao P, et al. Evaluation of a personalized, web-based decision aid for lung cancer screening. Am J Prev Med 2015;49(6):e125–9.
21. Mazzone PJ, Tenenbaum A, Seeley M, et al. Impact of a lung cancer screening counseling and shared decision-making visit. Chest 2017;151(3):572–8.
22. Leng J, Lui F, Gany F. Chinese livery drivers' perspectives on adapting a community health worker intervention to facilitate lung cancer screening. J Health Care Poor Underserved 2022;33(1):332–48.
23. Bouchard EG, Saad-Harfouche FG, Clark N, et al. Adapting community educational programs during the covid-19 pandemic: comparing the feasibility and efficacy of a lung cancer screening educational intervention by mode of delivery. J Cancer Educ 2022;1–9 [published online ahead of print, 2022 Jul 15].
24. Williams LB, Looney SW, Joshua T, et al. Promoting community awareness of lung cancer screening among disparate populations: results of the cancer-community awareness access research and education project. Cancer Nurs 2021;44(2):89–97.
25. Kathuria H, Gunawan A, Spring M, et al. Hospitalization as an opportunity to engage underserved individuals in shared decision-making for lung cancer screening: results from two randomized pilot trials. Cancer Causes Control 2022;33(11):1373–80.
26. Sakoda LC, Meyer MA, Chawla N, et al. Effectiveness of a patient education class to enhance knowledge about lung cancer screening: a quality

improvement evaluation. J Cancer Educ 2020;35(5): 897–904.

27. Fung LC, Nguyen KH, Stewart SL, et al. Impact of a cancer education seminar on knowledge and screening intent among Chinese Americans: Results from a randomized, controlled, community-based trial. Cancer 2018;124(Suppl 7):1622–30.

28. Adams SJ, Stone E, Baldwin DR, et al. Lung cancer screening [published online ahead of print, 2022 Dec 20]. Lancet 2022. https://doi.org/10.1016/S0140-6736(22)01694-4. S0140-6736(22)01694-4.

29. Crosbie PAJ, Gabe R, Simmonds I, et al. Participation in community-based lung cancer screening: the Yorkshire Lung Screening Trial. Eur Respir J 2022;60(5):2200483.

30. Dickson JL, Hall H, Horst C, et al, SUMMIT Consortium. Telephone risk-based eligibility assessment for low-dose CT lung cancer screening. Thorax 2022;77(10):1036–40.

31. Percac-Lima S, Ashburner JM, Rigotti NA, et al. Patient navigation for lung cancer screening among current smokers in community health centers a randomized controlled trial. Cancer Med 2018;7(3): 894–902.

32. Crosbie PA, Balata H, Evison M, et al. allmplementing lung cancer screening: baseline results from a community-based 'Lung Health Check' pilot in deprived areas of. ManchesterThorax 2019;74: 405–9.

33. Chiarantano RS, Vazquez FL, Franco A, et al. Implementation of an integrated lung cancer prevention and screening program using a mobile computed tomography (CT) Unit in Brazil. Cancer Control 2022;29. 10732748221121385.

34. Bartlett EC, Kemp SV, Ridge CA, et al, West London Lung Screening Collaboration Group. Baseline Results of the West London lung cancer screening pilot study - Impact of mobile scanners and dual risk model utilisation. Lung Cancer 2020;148:12–9.

35. Hochheimer CJ, Sabo RT, Tong ST, et al. Practice, clinician, and patient factors associated with the adoption of lung cancer screening. J Med Screen 2021;28(2):158–62.

36. Lerman C, Daly M, Sands C, et al. Mammography adherence and psychological distress among women at risk for breast cancer. J Natl Cancer Inst 1993;85(13):1074–80.

37. Champion VL, Monahan PO, Springston JK, et al. Measuring mammography and breast cancer beliefs in African American women. J Health Psychol 2008;13(6):827–37.

38. Bukowska-Durawa A, Luszczynska A. Cervical cancer screening and psychosocial barriers perceived by patients. A systematic review. Contemp Oncol 2014;18(3):153–9.

39. Bergamo C, Lin JJ, Smith C, et al. Evaluating beliefs associated with late-stage lung cancer presentation in minorities. J Thorac Oncol 2013;8(1):12–8.

40. Williams LB, Shelton BJ, Gomez ML, et al. Using implementation science to disseminate a lung cancer screening education intervention through community health workers. J Community Health 2021; 46(1):165–73.

Access to Lung Cancer Screening

Rian M. Hasson, MD[a,b,c], Connor J. Bridges, BS[b], Richard J. Curley, DrPH[d],
Loretta Erhunmwunsee, MD[d,e],*

KEYWORDS

- Low-dose chest computed tomography • Lung cancer screening barriers
- Non-small cell lung cancer • Health disparities

KEY POINTS

- Rural and racial/ethnic minority communities experience higher risk and mortality from lung cancer.
- Rural and racial/ethnic minority communities have lower rates of lung cancer screening (LCS).
- There are numerous barriers that marginalized communities face that limit access to LCS.
- Barriers to LCS are multilevel and include patient, provider, and system-level barriers.

INTRODUCTION

Lung cancer is the leading cause of cancer death among men and women in the United States, accounting for more deaths than colon, breast, and prostate cancers combined.[1] The American Cancer Society estimates that approximately 236,000 patients were diagnosed in 2022, with an estimated 130,000 (55%) cases resulting in death.[1] Treatment efforts at the earliest stage have proven most promising. Hence, studies designed to understand and standardize the benefits of lung cancer screening (LCS) are vital. Unfortunately, there remain significant barriers to accessing LCS, especially in rural and racial/ethnic minority communities. These marginalized communities already experience higher risk and mortality from lung cancer, thus the decrease in access to LCS only worsens lung cancer outcome disparities.

Early screening efforts primarily utilized chest x-rays, which were not convincingly shown to reduce mortality. Even in the early 2000s, no organization recommended routine LCS for either the general or the at-risk populations.[2] However, in 2011, data from the National Lung Screening Trial (NLST), a multi-institutional randomized controlled trial of 53,454 patients, formally demonstrated the utility of LCS by comparing low-dose computed tomography (LDCT) with chest x-ray.[3] They reported a *20% lung-specific mortality reduction*, and *a 6.7% overall mortality reduction in a high-risk cohort that underwent LDCT*.[3] As a result of these findings, many professional organizations published guidelines recommending annual screening for "high-risk" patients defined as those (1) aged 55 to 80 years, (2) with at least a 30 pack-year smoking history, (3) who are current or former smokers who have quit in the last 15 years.[4–9] Despite replication of these results,[10] and recent updates to United States Preventative Services Task Force (USPSTF) guidelines that include decreasing the age of eligibility to 50 from 55 years and pack-years to 20 from 30,[11] *LCS remains underutilized, especially in rural, racial/ethnic minority and underserved populations.*[12,13]

[a] Department of Surgery, Section of Thoracic Surgery, Dartmouth-Hitchcock Medical Center, 1 Medical Center Drive, Lebanon, NH 03756, USA; [b] The Geisel School of Medicine at Dartmouth, 1 Rope Ferry Rd, Hanover, NH 03755, USA; [c] The Dartmouth Institute of Health Policy and Clinical Practice, Williamson Translational Research Building, Level 51 Medical Center Drive Lebanon, NH 03756, USA; [d] Department of Surgery, City of Hope Comprehensive Cancer Center, 1500 East Duarte Road, Duarte, CA 91010, USA; [e] Department of Population Sciences, City of Hope Comprehensive Cancer Center, Duarte, CA, 91010, USA
* Corresponding author. Department of Surgery, City of Hope Comprehensive Cancer Center, 1500 East Duarte Road, Duarte, CA 91010.
E-mail address: LorettaE@coh.org

Thorac Surg Clin 33 (2023) 353–363
https://doi.org/10.1016/j.thorsurg.2023.03.003
1547-4127/23/© 2023 Elsevier Inc. All rights reserved.

The reasons for LCS underuse in marginalized communities are multifactorial and include systemic, patient, and provider roadblocks that have been hard to overcome (**Fig. 1**). As a result, less than 6% of qualifying high-risk patients participates in LCS,[14] compared with ~70% participation with breast and colon cancer-screening efforts.[15] Although breast and colon cancer screening efforts have benefited from provider education and patient marketing initiatives to increase awareness, to date, there have been very few large-scale LCS provider education or patient marketing campaigns to encourage provider and/or patient self-referrals to screening programs or improve levels of provider and patient knowledge regarding screening. Even though targeted screening based upon risk stratification has been shown to increase LCS uptake (with 80% of lives saved by targeting the highest at risk[16]), underserved populations continue to experience inequitable access to these targeted screening initiatives and LCS programs, which further contributes to the health disparities seen throughout the United States. Furthermore, a disproportionate number of eligible patients are either not referred, or do not follow-through with screening, which leads to excess and avoidable deaths each year. Recruitment and enrollment numbers in underserved populations (including rural and racial/ethnic minority groups) are even more discouraging, and although the reasons for this are likely also multifactorial, access to accredited facilities has historically been one of

the most common barriers to participation.[17–19] Hence, *there is a need to improve access and decrease the risk for low engagement to address this public health dilemma and improve uptake for eligible populations.*

Patient-Level Barriers

The barriers to LCS access are numerous. Even when screening resources are available, several patient-related hurdles persist. Commonly reported obstacles faced by rural and underserved populations include (1) limited knowledge of LCS, (2) a lack of information and unclear recommendations from health-care providers, (3) patient stigma often encountered from medical providers or the general public, and (4) unavailability of transportation.[20]

Decreased knowledge and education
Even though historically excluded groups (ie, racial, ethnic-minority individuals and those of low socioeconomic status [SES]) have higher risk and mortality from lung cancer, they face many barriers accessing potentially life-saving LCS. One important barrier is decreased knowledge regarding the tool. Although many patients nationwide are unfamiliar with LCS[19]—with up to 80% of LCS-eligible smokers having never heard of it[21]—racial and ethnic minorities seem to have even lower LCS knowledge and education.[22] A lack of knowledge and education may result from many factors, including decreased communication with primary care physicians (PCPs) about the existence of the annual LDCT guideline or its benefits.[23] This

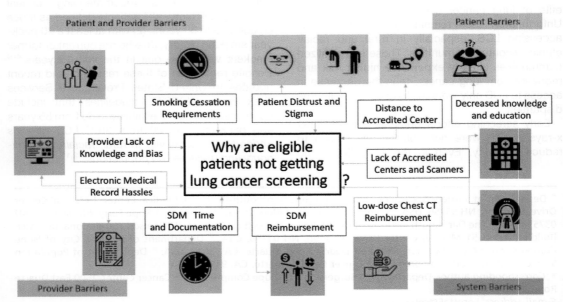

Fig. 1. Conceptual model describing barriers to LCS. Possible factors include institutional, financial, patient and provider obstacles that prevent participation in LCS. SDM, shared decision making.

decrease in communication leads to an unawareness of this important component of early detection and the patient's reluctance to screen even if the individual hears about the guideline in another venue (eg, social media, brochure in another health-care facility, and so forth).[24] Several studies have demonstrated that patients generally have a poor understanding of the risks and benefits of LCS[25–27] and rely on health-care professionals to address these knowledge gaps. Specific studies have shown that patients with lower education were less likely to understand why they were referred to LCS.[28] This may be because LCS education has several components, including the benefits of screening (both from a diagnostic, staging and outcome perspectives), the need to continue screening, tobacco cessation recommendations, and the potential costs associated with further workup of positive scans. Despite the LCS discussion complexity, when patients were educated on LCS, they were more willing to screen.[29]

Another patient-level barrier to LCS may decrease in appropriate lung cancer risk perception in marginalized communities. Although studies have found that risk perception is linked to willingness to undergo LCS,[30,31] motivation to screen is not static and can change overtime.[31] For instance, patients with a higher perceived risk of lung cancer are more likely to get LCS.[32] In contrast, patients that perceive themselves as healthy (have lower perceived risk) are less likely to undergo screening.[20] However, Latinx patients were more likely to think that NSCLC could be prevented and were less worried about developing NSCLC but were more likely to desire screening once informed.[29] Thus, lung cancer risk perception seems to affect the utilization in some communities but appropriate education may overcome this barrier.

More specifically, when it comes to educating patients, it is important to counsel on the reasons for LCS, how LCS works, and the need to continue with routine screening as with other screening protocols. One study at a rural, quaternary, academic institution reported a screening completion rate of only 22.6% among eligible patients who had their lung cancers operated on.[33] This suggests that if we are able to screen more patients, it is vital that they understand the importance of screening maintenance in order to decrease the high levels of attrition seen with LCS nationwide. Thus, patients without initial positive findings will have future lung cancer detected as soon as possible.

Patient distrust and stigma
In addition, a lack of trust in health-care providers can prevent screening.[19] Patient distrust in doctors[34] and the medical system[35] were negatively

associated with the intention to learn about and uptake LDCT scan at the individual level. Additionally, some LCS-eligible patients may only trust their PCP and thus wish to discuss screening only with that provider.[36] Invitations from PCPs were perceived as more trustworthy than those from screening centers.[37] Although it is understandable that patients want to receive screening information from their PCP, this behavior may limit the screening of racial and ethnic minorities who may not have regular PCPs or may take advice from other providers, such as nurses and medical assistants.[38]

Smokers and those with lung cancer feel stigmatized at higher rates. Many individuals, especially those of low-SES backgrounds, perceive LCS and smoking as sources of stigma that may lower their engagement with screening.[39] Data has demonstrated that the diagnosis and treatment of lung cancer has tremendous psychosocial consequences,[40] and patients with lung cancer have the highest rate of cancer-associated suicide.[41] Although the benefits of "survivorship" (the focus on health of patients with cancer, from posttreatment until the end of life) are well studied,[42,43] there has been an unmet need to address the emotional stress associated with screening,[44–47] and what prevents eligible patients from participating. This highlights the importance of educational campaigns in high-risk and rural areas because higher patient motivation and a humanistic approach from clinicians to screening were found to be linked to a greater understanding of the purpose of screening and the consequences of its absence.

Distance to accredited center
Unsurprisingly, distance to a CT facility is inversely related to population density, suggesting inequitable access among rural populations.[48] Analysis has shown that the urban-rural classification of residence is the most important predictor of availability of a CT facility, even after controlling for sociodemographic differences.[49] Capacity limitations are also a concern, with a 2014 study finding 127 of 805 (16%) Health Service Areas (HSAs) in the United States have no radiologists.[50] Further, among HSAs that are projected to have a greater 25% increase in scan volume due to increased LCS, the mean number of radiologists is effectively zero: 0.0155 (**Fig. 2**).[50] Thus, inadequate distribution of resources leaves many of the most vulnerable, rural populations with decreased access to screening facilities. Examples include New Hampshire and Vermont, which were found to have decreased access to accredited screening programs in areas with the greatest rates of smoking.[51]

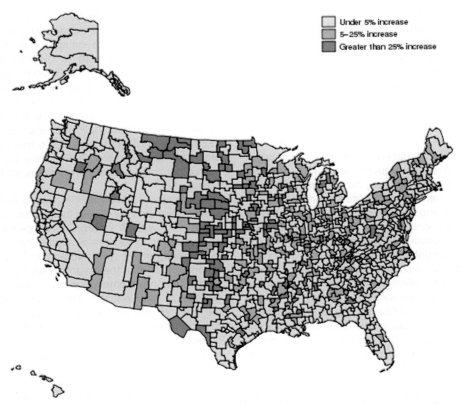

Fig. 2. Geographic distribution of demonstrating the projected radiologist capacity constraints. *From* Smieliaus-kas F, MacMahon H, Salgia R, Shih YC. Geographic variation in radiologist capacity and widespread implementation of lung cancer CT screening. J Med Screen. 2014;21(4):207-215.

Community outreach using a mobile LDCT unit was found to have detection and treatment rates consistent with the NLST.[52] Thus, mobile units are a promising solution to provide geographically isolated patients with access to LCS. However, the research group conducting the intervention described having to build the first LDCT mobile unit in the United States, despite publishing their article in 2020.[52] This underscores the lack of progress made in developing catchment initiatives aimed at remedying the stark geographic barriers to access and also limits the future reproducibility of these efforts, given the high costs often associated with these endeavors.

Social determinants of health

Cost is another barrier faced by racial minorities and underserved communities. Many individuals of low SES are uninsured or underinsured, preventing them from obtaining annual LCS.[53] A nationwide study that investigated challenges to LCS implementation at Federal Qualified Health Centers (FQHCs) found that the most significant barriers reported by individual facilities are

patients' lack of insurance, challenges obtaining prior insurance authorization, and coverage denials.[54] Moreover, Medicaid does not universally cover LCS, which may further affect LCS utilization in marginalized groups. Furthermore, some states have not adopted the Medicaid expansion, which leaves many low-income racial and ethnic minorities without coverage for LCS. In addition, poor communication regarding potential future patient costs of LCS has presented significant problems.[55] What to expect from a cost perspective for additional imaging and needed procedures represents a real fear for patients and is often overestimated given a lack of data.[56]

Additionally, in rural and less populated areas, having a reliable form of transportation to a screening appointment persists as a significant barrier to uptake (**Fig. 3**). A recent review estimates that in 2017, a lack of available transport caused 5.8 million patients in the United States to delay their medical care, an increase from the 4.8 million in 1997.[57] Rural residence is an independent risk factor for high travel mileage and time to access care, even after controlling for other variables.[58]

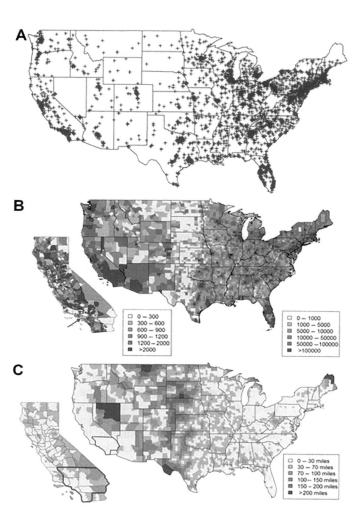

Fig. 3. Tobacco users in the United States and driving distance to an ACR 5 accredited facility. (A) Geographically coded locations of ACR-accredited CT facilities in the United States (n 5 6923). (B) Distribution of tobacco cigarette smokers in the United States. (C) Distance (by car) to the nearest ACR-accredited CT facility. (From Tailor TD, Choudhury KR, Tong BC, Christensen JD, Sosa JA, Rubin GD. Geographic Access to CT for Lung Cancer Screening: A Census Tract-Level Analysis of Cigarette Smoking in the United States and Driving Distance to a CT Facility. J Am Coll Radiol. 2019;16(1):15-23.)

This highlights the need for transportation options, which, beyond a personal vehicle, are scarce in rural areas given the low population densities and the resulting lack of public transportation options. Supporting this idea, an effort to increase health-care access through a free transportation program showed positive effects on physical, mental, and financial health of patients,[59] and this could likely be applied to an LCS initiative.

Provider-level barriers

Provider knowledge and bias

Provider education, awareness, and beliefs can prevent the identification of patients and LCS referrals. Provider limitations extend beyond inadequate provision of information and recommendations. More than half of PCPs are unaware of USPSTF recommendations for LCS with LDCT.[60] Knowledge of available resources is also an issue because almost half of PCPs are unaware that an LCS service exists in their geographic area.[6] Beliefs and barriers that have been reported include the perception that there is a low detection rate with LDCT, a lack of mortality reduction, the lack of EMR notification, high rates of patient refusal, high costs to patients, and harmful effects of radiation exposure, among others.[53,61,62] In a study of Los Angeles providers, only 37% thought they could adequately identify patients for LCS, and 69% thought insurance plans did not cover LCS.[53] Coughlin and colleagues found lower levels of awareness among physicians in 3 different health-care settings (a university tertiary care center, a public safety net hospital, and 3 community hospitals) because only 6.2% (of the 96 providers who responded) correctly identified all of the 6 CMS LDCT eligibility criteria when presented with 3 incorrect criteria.[62] They also found that minimal increases in provider knowledge (a one-point increase on a survey scale) was associated with a 13% increase in the likelihood that an LDCT would be ordered for eligible patients. In another study, only 47% of respondents knew that the USPSTF recommended LCS.[61] In the study by Akhtar and colleagues, almost half of the providers agreed that they might not make referrals because "LCS is too expensive for our healthcare system" (46%) or because "patient(s) cannot afford or lack adequate coverage for LCS" (46%).[53] Furthermore, providers indicated that several factors would influence their decision to refer patients for LCS, including a lack of clarity on the benefit of LCS (69%), not having time to discuss the risks and benefits of LCS (77%), and the high risks of LCS (77%). The less-than-ideal provider knowledge of LCS potentially limits opportunities for improved patient understanding. This, combined with the low motivation of underserved rural and racial populations that are burdened by systemic barriers preventing access to LCS, leads to underutilization of LDCT and negative downstream consequences for these communities.

When it comes to the workforce needed to maintain LCS and the downstream implications for positive scans, it is important to note that the median wait time for lung cancer surgery already stood at 35 days in 2003 to 2005, up from 25 in 1995 to 1997 and is likely to have only increased since then.[63] Increased implementation of LDCT screening programs will increase surgical volume.[64] So even if we are able to get patients screened, the shortage of cardiothoracic surgeons, coupled with the decreased proportion of physicians who live in rural areas compared with the general population,[65] will lead to further decreases in access and contribute to mortality if not addressed alongside primary care issues. In 2018, one projection described an expected 61% increase in cardiothoracic surgery cases alongside a 121% increase in per-surgeon workload by 2035.[66]

Electronic medical record hassles

The uptake of Electronic Medical Records (EMRs) has increased rapidly in the United States. The EMR was expected to improve the accuracy of information and support clinical decision-making.[67] Many providers recognize the importance of using EMRs for documenting smoking history.[68–70] For instance, by collecting key smoking exposure data, such as packs smoked per day and years smoked,[68] providers can use EMRs to identify high-risk patients and refer them to LCS.[68,69] However, growing research reveals inadequate and unreliable smoking history data that may lead to low rates of LCS.

A recent study by Kukhareva and colleagues assessing the accuracy of smoking history in the EMR found that there were significant errors throughout the EMR.[68] Of the 16,874 patient records, 80% had inaccuracies, including missing packs-per-day or years-smoked (42.7%), outdated data (25.1%), and missing years-quit date (17.4%).[68] In a study of 110 FQHCs, only 54% reported routinely documenting pack-year history in the EMR, and only 29% thought the documented smoking history to be "very accurate."[54] Inaccurate smoking history in EMR may reduce the LCS screening rate and lead to disparity in marginalized communities.

Shared decision-making time and documentation

Shared decision-making (SDM) is a feature unique to LCS that involves a thorough discussion of benefits and risks mandated to occur between providers and patients before ordering an LDCT[5,56]; however, it has been a barrier to LCS referral and enrollment, for this exact reason. Comprehensive SDM is associated with a better understanding of LCS, reduced decisional conflict regarding screening choice, and increased likelihood to adhere to annual LCS guidelines.[57] Nevertheless, from a provider perspective, finding the time to complete the SDM has proven to be an arduous task with few resources available to relieve this burden placed on health-care clinicians. Recent analysis in *JAMA* demonstrated that physician knowledge and comfort was low, efforts were brief, observed quality of SDM was poor, and explanation of potential harms was frequently absent or misreported.[17]

Patient and Provider-Level Barriers

Smoking cessation requirement

Historically the misconception that screening-eligible patients need to cease tobacco use before screening, along with low patient motivation to know their lung cancer status, have posed a barrier to uptake. Previous marketing campaigns often touted the phrase, "You stopped smoking, now start screening,"[71] which perpetuated the idea that eligible patients had to stop smoking to screen for lung cancer (**Fig. 4**). Although tobacco cessation counseling is a required component of the SDM conversations, and quitting is highly recommended, the importance of screening even in the presence of continued tobacco use must not be undermined and much research has been done to combat the unfortunate consequences of these campaigns to increase the uptake. It is reassuring to know, that when patients do commit to tobacco cessation and are able to either decrease or stop smoking, they are more likely to screen as recommended.[72] Among a cohort of

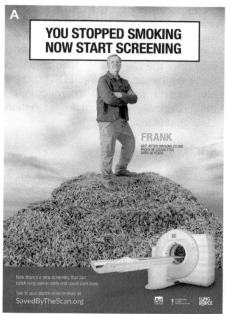
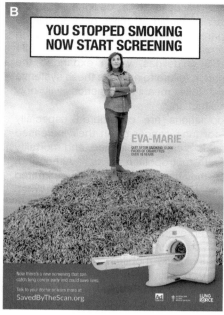

Fig. 4. "You stopped smoking, now start Screening" LCS marketing campaign. Although the advertisements 2(*A, B*) celebrate tobacco cessation, it implies screening is reserved for those that have quit and not for those that continue to smoke cigarettes. (*Courtesy of* Ad Council and American Lung Association's Saved By The Scan campaign.)

LCS-eligible patients, having quit smoking or currently smoking less than before was the only attitude, belief, or behavior shown to significantly differ between those who followed through with LDCT and those who ultimately decided to defer LDCT to a later date. As the authors concluded, the similarity in patient attitudes, beliefs, and behaviors between these 2 groups suggest that patient adherence to LCS likely depends on the practices of their PCPs to share information about tobacco use and cessation,[72] answer patient questions and concerns, and promote LCS as we know many patients often agree to screening based on provider recommendations. Additionally, the fact that while low motivation to know *the results* of screening was cited as a further barrier, high motivation stemming from provider conversations was found to facilitate the likelihood of pursuing lung[73] and other cancer screenings.[74]

System-Level Barriers

Lack of accredited centers and scanners
Geographic disparities in LCS have been well documented, with variations both within and between states. At a national level, LCS has suffered from a paucity of successful targeted efforts designed to increase uptake. Although possible solutions have included modeling strategies to optimize cancer screenings to increase compliance,[75] none of these

ideas has gained serious traction or has been recognized with much significance in the United States.

Full access to LCS registry facilities is only available in 63% of counties in the United States, with 19% having partial access and 18% having no access.[76] There is a general pattern of increased access in eastern states, with greater in-state variation observed in central and western parts of the country (see **Fig. 3**).[76] The impact of Medicaid expansion on LCS is also noteworthy in the discussion of system-related barriers. To date, 38 states have adopted Medicaid expansion.[77] The remaining 12, most of which have an average poverty rate of 12% to 15%, are yet to expand Medicaid.[78] Consequently, many residents of these states may lack access to preventive services guaranteed under Medicaid expansion.[79] A 2017 study of the geographic availability of LDCT in the United States found that across all states, 14.9% of individuals aged 55 to 79 years did not have access to a designated screening center within 30 miles, and 28% did not have access within a 30-minute drive. In 4 states (North Dakota, South Dakota, Montana, and Wyoming), 66% to 86% did not have access to LDCT within 30 miles.[54] Two states (South Dakota and Wyoming) have not adopted Medicaid expansion. These patterns of disparity were more salient in rural areas as rural residents were less likely to have access to a designated LDCT screening center within 30 miles or a 30-minute drive compared with urban residents. Although these patterns were found before the new 2021 USPSTF LCS guidelines, which expanded the eligibility criteria, failure to address these systemic barriers and take meaningful action will only worsen the situation.

Rural populations are considered especially "high-risk" for lung cancer given their increased rates of smoking, cancer incidence, and mortality compared with metropolitan areas.[80] Although it is imperative they have access to LCS, estimated uptake is much lower in rural cohorts.[14] When looking at the conceptual model for the reasons screening is less effective (see **Fig. 1**), accessibility continues to represent a tremendous known barrier. However, there is evidence to support novel interventions including mobile screening units to address this population-based obstacle.[20,81] Nevertheless, in-depth examination of downstream barriers and possible risk factors for low patient engagement in interventions with mobile screening units is needed to understand how to address high-attrition rates.

Low-dose chest computed tomography and shared decision-making reimbursement
Limited resources and low-reimbursement rates are also potential explanations for the limited number of LCS catchment programs. Challenges in implementing LCS clinics and SDM, a key component of LCS, include reliance on grant funding, difficulty maintaining the necessary resources, and limited staff to deliver SDM.[82] Low reimbursements for LCS and SDM provision relative to other services impose financial limitations on their widespread implementation, often leaving grant or industry funding as the only viable option. The low reimbursement from SDM, low reimbursement for low-dose CT scan interpretations, and EMR hassles can greatly inhibit a clinician's ability to consistently promote and recommend screening. Because most other cancer screenings merely require an order/referral for either the scan, test, or procedure, the more complicated LCS process contributes to the very low 6% uptake in LCS compared with greater than 70% uptake in other screening modalities.

Other systemic barriers include preauthorization requirements and limited resources in health-care centers that serve socioeconomically disadvantaged individuals. A study that investigated issues faced by FQHCs in the implementation of LCS in low-resource settings found that among 258 FQHCs sampled, less than half (23%) reported offering some LCS, and 58% reported issues with preauthorization.[54] The study also found that only 12% reported that leadership had allocated resources, and only 12% prioritized LCS. Although this study was conducted in 2016 (a year after the Centers for Medicare and Medicaid Services began covering LDCT screening), one can expect peripheral improvement based on the historically slow uptake of national health-care guidelines.

SUMMARY

LCS utilization is remarkably low even though lung cancer is the number one cancer killer. There are numerous barriers that limit access of those at highest risk to the life-saving screening modality. Patient, provider, and system-level hurdles are particularly troublesome for those at highest risk, including racial and ethnic minorities and those within rural and low-SES communities. It is critical that we acknowledge and intervene on these challenges so that outcomes are improved for all groups.

CLINICS CARE POINTS

- LCS efforts should include structured and tailored educational campaigns in high-risk and rural areas that target increases in provider and patient awareness of lung cancer risk, LCS guidelines, and the benefits of LCS.
- There should be universal efforts to improve the accuracy of smoking exposure data in EMRs.
- Both smoking cessation discussions and LCS SDM efforts should be better supported with increased reimbursement and personnel assistance.

DISCLOSURE

L. Erhunmwunsee reports a relationship with AstraZeneca Pharmaceuticals LP that includes board membership, funding grants, and speaking and lecture fees. L. Erhunmwunsee reports a relationship with Gilead Oncology that includes speaking and lecture fees.

REFERENCES

1. American Cancer Society. Key statistics for lung cancer. American Cancer Society; 2019.
2. Smith RA, von Eschenbach AC, Wender R, et al. American Cancer Society guidelines for the early

detection of cancer: update of early detection guidelines for prostate, colorectal, and endometrial cancers. Also: update 2001–testing for early lung cancer detection. CA Cancer J Clin 2001;51(1): 38–75. quiz 77-80.

3. National Lung Screening Trial Research T, Aberle DR, Adams AM, et al. Reduced lung-cancer mortality with low-dose computed tomographic screening. N Engl J Med 2011;365(5):395–409.

4. American Lung Association. Providing Guidance on Lung Cancer Screening. The American Lung Association Interim Report on Lung Cancer Screening. Available at: http://www.lung.org/lung-disease/lung-cancer/lung-cancer-screening-guidelines/lung-cancer-screening.pdf. Accessed 15 October, 2018.

5. Bach PB, Mirkin JN, Oliver TK, et al. Benefits and harms of CT screening for lung cancer: a systematic review. JAMA 2012;307(22):2418–29.

6. Detterbeck FC, Mazzone PJ, Naidich DP, et al. Screening for lung cancer: Diagnosis and management of lung cancer, 3rd ed: American College of Chest Physicians evidence-based clinical practice guidelines. Chest 2013;143(5 Suppl):e78S–92S.

7. Jaklitsch MT, Jacobson FL, Austin JH, et al. The American Association for Thoracic Surgery guidelines for lung cancer screening using low-dose computed tomography scans for lung cancer survivors and other high-risk groups. J Thorac Cardiovasc Surg 2012;144(1):33–8.

8. National Comprehensive Cancer Network. NCCN Clinical Practice Guidelines in Oncology: Lung Cancer Screening. Version 1. 2013. Published 2013. Accessed October 15, 2018.

9. Wender R, Fontham ETH, Barrera E Jr, et al. American Cancer Society lung cancer screening guidelines. CA A Cancer J Clin 2013;63(2):106–17.

10. de Koning HJ, van der Aalst CM, de Jong PA, et al. Reduced Lung-Cancer Mortality with Volume CT Screening in a Randomized Trial. N Engl J Med 2020;382(6):503–13.

11. U.S. Preventive Services Task Force. Final Recommnedation Statement – Lung Cancer: Screening. https://www.uspreventiveservicestaskforce.org/uspstf/recommendation/lung-cancer-screening. Published 2021. Updated March 09, 2021. Accessed 1 August, 2021.

12. Rivera MP, Katki HA, Tanner NT, et al. Addressing Disparities in Lung Cancer Screening Eligibility and Healthcare Access. An Official American Thoracic Society Statement. Am J Respir Crit Care Med 2020;202(7):e95–112.

13. Sosa E, D'Souza G, Akhtar A, et al. Racial and socioeconomic disparities in lung cancer screening in the United States: A systematic review. CA Cancer J Clin 2021;71(4):299–314.

14. Atkins GT, Kim T, Munson J. Residence in Rural Areas of the United States and Lung Cancer Mortality. Disease Incidence, Treatment Disparities, and Stage-Specific Survival. Ann Am Thorac Soc 2017;14(3):403–11.

15. U.S. Centers for Disease Control and Prevention. U.S. Cancer Statistics Data Visualization Tool. https://www.cdc.gov/cancer/colorectal/statistics/index.htm. Published 2021. Accessed 1 August, 2021.

16. Kumar V, Cohen JT, van Klaveren D, et al. Risk-Targeted Lung Cancer Screening: A Cost-Effectiveness Analysis. Ann Intern Med 2018;168(3):161–9.

17. Brenner AT, Malo TL, Margolis M, et al. Evaluating Shared Decision Making for Lung Cancer Screening. JAMA Intern Med 2018;178(10):1311–6.

18. Lewis JA, Chen H, Weaver KE, et al. Low Provider Knowledge Is Associated With Less Evidence-Based Lung Cancer Screening. J Natl Compr Canc Netw 2019;17(4):339–46.

19. Wang GX, Baggett TP, Pandharipande PV, et al. Barriers to Lung Cancer Screening Engagement from the Patient and Provider Perspective. Radiology 2019;290(2):278–87.

20. Schiffelbein JE, Carluzzo KL, Hasson RM, et al. Barriers, Facilitators, and Suggested Interventions for Lung Cancer Screening Among a Rural Screening-Eligible Population. J Prim Care Community Health 2020;11. 2150132720930544.

21. Raz DJ, Wu G, Nelson RA, et al. Perceptions and Utilization of Lung Cancer Screening Among Smokers Enrolled in a Tobacco Cessation Program. Clin Lung Cancer 2019;20(1):e115–22.

22. Carter-Harris L, Slaven JE Jr, Monahan PO, et al. Understanding lung cancer screening behavior: Racial, gender, and geographic differences among Indiana long-term smokers. Prev Med Rep 2018; 10:49–54.

23. Carter-Harris L, Tan AS, Salloum RG, et al. Patient-provider discussions about lung cancer screening pre- and post-guidelines: Health Information National Trends Survey (HINTS). Patient Educ Couns 2016;99(11):1772–7.

24. Wiener RS, Koppelman E, Bolton R, et al. Patient and Clinician Perspectives on Shared Decision-making in Early Adopting Lung Cancer Screening Programs: a Qualitative Study. J Gen Intern Med 2018;33(7):1035–42.

25. Sakoda LC, Meyer MA, Chawla N, et al. Effectiveness of a Patient Education Class to Enhance Knowledge about Lung Cancer Screening: a Quality Improvement Evaluation. J Cancer Educ 2020;35(5): 897–904.

26. Tan NQP, Nishi SPE, Lowenstein LM, et al. Impact of the shared decision-making process on lung cancer screening decisions. Cancer Med 2022;11(3):790–7.

27. Reuland DS, Cubillos L, Brenner AT, et al. A pre-post study testing a lung cancer screening decision aid in primary care. BMC Med Inform Decis Mak 2018; 18(1):5.

28. Hall DL, Lennes IT, Carr A, et al. Lung Cancer Screening Uncertainty among Patients Undergoing LDCT. Am J Health Behav 2018;42(1):69–76.

29. Percac-Lima S, Ashburner JM, Atlas SJ, et al. Barriers to and Interest in Lung Cancer Screening Among Latino and Non-Latino Current and Former Smokers. J Immigr Minor Health 2019;21(6):1313–24.

30. Quaife SL, Waller J, Dickson JL, et al. Psychological Targets for Lung Cancer Screening Uptake: A Prospective Longitudinal Cohort Study. J Thorac Oncol 2021;16(12):2016–28.

31. Gillespie C, Wiener RS, Clark JA. Patient Experience of Managing Adherence to Repeat Lung Cancer Screening. Journal of Patient Experience 2022;9. 23743735221126146.

32. See K, Manser R, Park ER, et al. The impact of perceived risk, screening eligibility and worry on preference for lung cancer screening: a cross-sectional survey. ERJ Open Res 2020;6(1).

33. Hasson RM, Phillips JD, Fay KA, et al. Lung Cancer Screening in a Surgical Lung Cancer Population: Analysis of a Rural, Quaternary, Academic Experience. J Surg Res 2021;262:14–20.

34. Jia Q, Chen H, Chen X, et al. Barriers to Low-Dose CT Lung Cancer Screening among Middle-Aged Chinese. Int J Environ Res Public Health 2020; 17(19).

35. Lei F, Lee E. Barriers to Lung Cancer Screening With Low-Dose Computed Tomography. Oncol Nurs Forum 2019;46(2):E60–71.

36. Simmons VN, Gray JE, Schabath MB, et al. High-risk community and primary care providers knowledge about and barriers to low-dose computed topography lung cancer screening. Lung cancer (Amsterdam, Netherlands) 2017;106:42–9.

37. Young B, Bedford L, Kendrick D, et al. Factors influencing the decision to attend screening for cancer in the UK: a meta-ethnography of qualitative research. J Public Health 2018;40(2):315–39.

38. Arnett MJ, Thorpe RJ Jr, Gaskin DJ, et al. Race, Medical Mistrust, and Segregation in Primary Care as Usual Source of Care: Findings from the Exploring Health Disparities in Integrated Communities Study. J Urban Health 2016;93(3):456–67.

39. Olson RE, Goldsmith L, Winter S, et al. Emotions and lung cancer screening: Prioritising a humanistic approach to care. Health Soc Care Community 2022;30(6):e5259–69.

40. Looijmans M, van Manen AS, Traa MJ, et al. Psychosocial consequences of diagnosis and treatment of lung cancer and evaluation of the need for a lung cancer specific instrument using focus group methodology. Support Care Cancer 2018;26(12):4177–85.

41. Rahouma M, Kamel M, Abouarab A, et al. Lung cancer patients have the highest malignancy-associated suicide rate in USA: a population-based analysis. Ecancermedicalscience 2018;12:859.

42. Berman AT, DeCesaris CM, Simone CB 2nd, et al. Use of Survivorship Care Plans and Analysis of Patient-Reported Outcomes in Multinational Patients With Lung Cancer. J Oncol Pract 2016;12(5):e527–35.

43. Sloan JA, Cheville AL, Liu H, et al. Impact of self-reported physical activity and health promotion behaviors on lung cancer survivorship. Health Qual Life Outcomes 2016;14:66.

44. Hamann HA, Ver Hoeve ES, Carter-Harris L, et al. Multilevel Opportunities to Address Lung Cancer Stigma across the Cancer Control Continuum. J Thorac Oncol 2018;13(8):1062–75.

45. Occhipinti S, Dunn J, O'Connell DL, et al. Lung Cancer Stigma across the Social Network: Patient and Caregiver Perspectives. J Thorac Oncol 2018; 13(10):1443–53.

46. Rose S, Boyes A, Kelly B, et al. Help-seeking behaviour in newly diagnosed lung cancer patients: Assessing the role of perceived stigma. Psycho Oncol 2018;27(9):2141–7.

47. Rose S, Kelly B, Boyes A, et al. Impact of Perceived Stigma in People Newly Diagnosed With Lung Cancer: A Cross-Sectional Analysis. Oncol Nurs Forum 2018;45(6):737–47.

48. Tailor TD, Choudhury KR, Tong BC, et al. Geographic Access to CT for Lung Cancer Screening: A Census Tract-Level Analysis of Cigarette Smoking in the United States and Driving Distance to a CT Facility. J Am Coll Radiol 2019;16(1):15–23.

49. Tailor TD, Tong BC, Gao J, et al. A Geospatial Analysis of Factors Affecting Access to CT Facilities: Implications for Lung Cancer Screening. J Am Coll Radiol 2019;16(12):1663–8.

50. Smieliauskas F, MacMahon H, Salgia R, et al. Geographic variation in radiologist capacity and widespread implementation of lung cancer CT screening. J Med Screen 2014;21(4):207–15.

51. Hasson RM, Fay KA, Phillips JD, et al. Rural barriers to early lung cancer detection: Exploring access to lung cancer screening programs in New Hampshire and Vermont. Am J Surg 2021;221(4):725–30.

52. Raghavan D, Wheeler M, Doege D, et al. Initial Results from Mobile Low-Dose Computerized Tomographic Lung Cancer Screening Unit: Improved Outcomes for Underserved Populations. Oncol 2020;25(5):e777–81.

53. Akhtar A, Sosa E, Castro S, et al. A Lung Cancer Screening Education Program Impacts both Referral Rates and Provider and Medical Assistant Knowledge at Two Federally Qualified Health Centers. Clin Lung Cancer 2022;23(4):356–63.

54. Zeliadt SB, Hoffman RM, Birkby G, et al. Challenges Implementing Lung Cancer Screening in Federally Qualified Health Centers. Am J Prev Med 2018; 54(4):568–75.

55. Scoggins JF, Fedorenko CR, Donahue SM, et al. Is distance to provider a barrier to care for medicaid

patients with breast, colorectal, or lung cancer? J Rural Health 2012;28(1):54–62.

56. Black WC. Importance of Individualized Decision Making for Lung Cancer Screening. Radiology 2018;289(1):225–6.

57. Wolfe MK, McDonald NC, Holmes GM. Transportation Barriers to Health Care in the United States: Findings From the National Health Interview Survey, 1997-2017. Am J Public Health 2020;110(6):815–22.

58. Probst JC, Laditka SB, Wang JY, et al. Effects of residence and race on burden of travel for care: cross sectional analysis of the 2001 US National Household Travel Survey. BMC Health Serv Res 2007;7:40.

59. Schwartz AJ, Richman AR, Scott M, et al. Increasing Access to Care for the Underserved: Voices of Riders, Drivers, & Staff of a Rural Transportation Program. Int J Environ Res Public Health 2022;19(20).

60. Raz DJ, Wu GX, Consunji M, et al. Perceptions and Utilization of Lung Cancer Screening Among Primary Care Physicians. J Thorac Oncol 2016; 11(11):1856–62.

61. Raz DJ, Wu GX, Consunji M, et al. The effect of primary care physician knowledge of lung cancer screening guidelines on perceptions and utilization of low-dose computed tomography. Clin Lung Cancer 2018;19(1):51–7.

62. Coughlin JM, Zang Y, Terranella S, et al. Understanding barriers to lung cancer screening in primary care. J Thorac Dis 2020;12(5):2536–44.

63. Bilimoria KY, Ko CY, Tomlinson JS, et al. Wait times for cancer surgery in the United States: trends and predictors of delays. Ann Surg 2011;253(4):779–85.

64. Hung YC, Tang EK, Wu YJ, et al. Impact of low-dose computed tomography for lung cancer screening on lung cancer surgical volume: The urgent need in health workforce education and training. Medicine (Baltim) 2021;100(32):e26901.

65. Staiger DO, Marshall SM, Goodman DC, et al. Association Between Having a Highly Educated Spouse and Physician Practice in Rural Underserved Areas. JAMA 2016;315(9):939–41.

66. Moffatt-Bruce S, Crestanello J, Way DP, et al. Providing cardiothoracic services in 2035: signs of trouble ahead. J Thorac Cardiovasc Surg 2018; 155(2):824–9.

67. Honavar SG. Electronic medical records - The good, the bad and the ugly. Indian J Ophthalmol 2020; 68(3):417–8.

68. Kukhareva PV, Caverly TJ, Li H, et al. Inaccuracies in electronic health records smoking data and a potential approach to address resulting underestimation in determining lung cancer screening eligibility. J Am Med Inform Assoc 2022;29(5):779–88.

69. Tarabichi Y, Kats DJ, Kaelber DC, et al. The Impact of Fluctuations in Pack-Year Smoking History in the Electronic Health Record on Lung Cancer Screening Practices. Chest 2018;153(2):575–8.

70. Modin HE, Fathi JT, Gilbert CR, et al. Pack-Year Cigarette Smoking History for Determination of Lung Cancer Screening Eligibility. Comparison of the Electronic Medical Record versus a Shared Decision-making Conversation. Ann Am Thorac Soc 2017;14(8):1320–5.

71. American Lung Association. LuCA National Training Network Resource Library. Available at: https://luca training.org/services/resource-library/you-stopped-smoking-now-start-screening. Accessed 1 January, 2023.

72. Duong DK, Shariff-Marco S, Cheng I, et al. Patient and primary care provider attitudes and adherence towards lung cancer screening at an academic medical center. Prev Med Rep 2017;6:17–22.

73. Holman A, Kross E, Crothers K, et al. Patient Perspectives on Longitudinal Adherence to Lung Cancer Screening. Chest 2022;162(1):230–41.

74. Kindratt TB, Atem F, Dallo FJ, et al. The Influence of Patient-Provider Communication on Cancer Screening. J Patient Exp 2020;7(6):1648–57.

75. Taksler GB, Peterse EFP, Willems I, et al. Modeling Strategies to Optimize Cancer Screening in USPSTF Guideline-Noncompliant Women. JAMA Oncol 2021; 7(6):885–94.

76. Sahar L, Douangchai Wills VL, Liu KK, et al. Using Geospatial Analysis to Evaluate Access to Lung Cancer Screening in the United States. Chest 2021;159(2):833–44.

77. KFF. Status of State Medicaid Expansion Decisions: Interactive Map | KFF. Available at: https://www.kff. org/medicaid/issue-brief/status-of-state-medicaid-expansion-decisions-interactive-map/. Accessed 5 January, 2023.

78. AGRICULTURE USDO. Poverty. Available at: https:// data.ers.usda.gov/reports.aspx?ID=17826. Accessed 5 January, 2023.

79. Association AL. Medicaid Expansion and Lung Cancer. Available at: https://www.lung.org/getmedia/ 13a5c27f-c3de-4b57-af22-bee6e578831c/Medicaid-Expansion-and-LCS-One-Pager-2020-Final(1). Accessed January 5, 2023.

80. Odahowski CL, Zahnd WE, Eberth JM. Challenges and Opportunities for Lung Cancer Screening in Rural America. J Am Coll Radiol 2019;16(4 Pt B):590–5.

81. Vang S, Margolies LR, Jandorf L. Mobile Mammography Participation Among Medically Underserved Women: A Systematic Review. Prev Chronic Dis 2018;15:E140.

82. Alishahi Tabriz A, Neslund-Dudas C, Turner K, et al. How Health-Care Organizations Implement Shared Decision-making When It Is Required for Reimbursement: The Case of Lung Cancer Screening. Chest 2021;159(1):413–25.

Advancing Health Equity in Lung Cancer Screening and the Role of Humanomics

Zachary Hartley-Blossom, MD, MBA[a],*, Alejandra Cardona-Del Valle, MD[b],
Claudia Muns-Aponte, BS[b], Neha Udayakumar, MD[c],
Ruth C. Carlos, MD, MS[d], Efren J. Flores, MD[a],*

KEYWORDS

- Humanomics • Lung cancer • Lung cancer screening • Health equity • Social genomics

KEY POINTS

- Systemic inequities and discrimination can affect gene expressivity and may predispose individuals to cancer development, according to Humanomics.
- Lung cancer screening can decrease disparities in morbidity and mortality; however, despite the recent expansion of the US Preventative Services Task Force screening inclusion criteria, only a small fraction of eligible patients undergo screening.
- To expand access to lung cancer screening, we must acknowledge and address the multifactorial individual, provider, and system-level barriers that disproportionately affect certain communities.

INTRODUCTION

Lung cancer (LC) remains the leading cause of cancer-specific mortality in the United States despite numerous advances in treatment and early detection. In 2022, there were an estimated 254,850 new cases and 135,360 deaths alone.[1] Although LC impacts all races, ethnicities, and communities, disparities in LC outcomes still exist. Factors leading to these disparities include but are not limited to medical and sociodemographic factors such as language, stigma surrounding tobacco use, LC diagnosis and treatment, health literacy, access to smoking cessation resources, and other social determinants of health (SDoH).[2,3] The combination of these factors and their impact on the individual can be termed social genomics or humanomics.

LC screening (LCS) offers a unique opportunity to decrease existing LC disparities among those communities disproportionately bearing the burden of increased morbidity and mortality from LC. However, despite the documented benefits of LCS in reducing mortality, only a small fraction of eligible patients undergo screening, and an even smaller proportion of those from minority communities.[4] Over the last several years, during the ongoing COVID-19 pandemic, health disparities among racial/ethnic minority communities were exacerbated as resources were redirected to the immediate need to deal with the pandemic.[4,5] Although the long-term impact of this, including the delaying of routine medical care and screening, is not yet known, failure to develop targeted approaches for these communities will likely widen the disparities in LCS and, subsequently, LC mortality.[5]

The recent update on the US Preventative Services Task Force (USPSTF) broadened inclusion criteria by lowering the required age (50 years from 55 years) and the required smoking history

[a] Division of Thoracic Imaging, Department of Radiology, Massachusetts General Hospital, 55 Fruit Street, Boston, MA 02114, USA; [b] Department of Radiology, University of Puerto Rico School of Medicine, Rio Piedras Medical Center Americo Miranda Avenue, San Juan, 00936, Puerto Rico; [c] Department of Radiology, Massachusetts General Hospital, 55 Fruit Street, Boston, MA 02114, USA; [d] Department of Radiology, University of Michigan, 1500 East Medical Center Drive, Ste C21, Ann Arbor, MI 48109, USA
* Corresponding authors.
E-mail addresses: zhartley-blossom@mgh.harvard.edu; zhartley@umich.edu (Z.H.-B.); ejflores@mgh.harvard.edu (E.J.F.)

Thorac Surg Clin 33 (2023) 365–373
https://doi.org/10.1016/j.thorsurg.2023.04.007
1547-4127/23/© 2023 Elsevier Inc. All rights reserved.

(20 pack-years from 30 pack-years).[6] In addition, there has been an increased attention to cancer outcomes and prevention from the highest levels of government with the revitalization of Cancer Moonshot and the goals of reducing cancer mortality by 50% over the next 25 years.[7]

As inclusion criteria for LCS and focus on cancer outcomes broaden, our evaluation needs to broaden to factors outside of the individual, both macroscopically and microscopically. This includes an assessment at the societal system level as well as the cellular level. Linking these topics with humanomics requires an acceptance and understanding that external inequities and stressors can directly affect an individual's genetics. For example, increased external stress, either by racial segregation, overt hostility, or heightened vigilance, induces an increased level of ambient stress.[8] This increased ambient stress may lead to downstream consequences, including the upregulation of inflammatory cascades and the creation of a pro-oncotic environment.

These revelations offer a unique opportunity to reexamine our LCS engagement practices. The purpose of this article is to discuss a framework for increasing LCS uptake within racial and ethnic minority communities by improving awareness, opportunities, and participation in LCS by examining both upstream societal structures and individual experiences using a modified socioecological model including humanomics. Understanding these effects' intersection is crucial in reducing disparities in LCS and LC mortality.

LUNG CANCER SCREENING AWARENESS
Barriers

At the individual level, some barriers to LCS awareness include unawareness of the new USPSTF and Centers for Medicare and Medicaid Services (CMS) recommendations and cost (or lack thereof) among payors. In addition, there may be uncertainty about available local LCS programs in their community. Finally, there can be a lack of culturally appropriate information, or the information is delivered at an inappropriate health literacy level (Fig. 1).[9–11]

At the provider level, there may be uncertainty related to new USPSTF and CMS recommendations, insurance coverage, or identifying newly eligible patients under these guidelines.[10–12] Additional barriers include unfamiliarity of appropriate centers to refer patients when accounting for insurance coverage, or where to refer patients in the case of an abnormal LCS finding.[11] This may be even more prevalent in relatively more resource dearth communities when it comes to available

pulmonologists, surgeons, and oncologists.[11] Finally, there may be skepticism surrounding the generalizability of LCS, given that the trials touting the survival benefit of LCS primarily recruited White, Non-Hispanic patients from higher socioeconomic statuses relative to the general population.[11]

From a community and systems perspective, information about LCS is often not tailored to the language or culture of the surrounding communities. In addition, failing to understand how to use social media best to communicate this information limits community outreach.[13,14] Finally, electronic medical records (EMRs) are not optimized to identify eligible patients and automatically notify patients or providers of their LCS-eligible status (see Fig. 1).

Facilitators/Opportunities

At the individual level, the primary opportunity is centered on appropriate, patient-centered educational content. Educational materials via conventional and social media channels need to be culturally tailored, at a proper health literacy level, and in commonly used languages within the community served by the institution. This information must alleviate some patient-level concerns, including information about available sites, insurance coverage, and eligibility criteria. In addition, the educational material needs to be curated and delivered to foster patient engagement while increasing familiarity and reducing stigma with the LCS process.[11] Prior studies have demonstrated that using social media can be an effective way to increase LCS awareness and engagement.[15] This requires an intimate understanding of the surrounding communities because the best avenues/channels for communication are likely to vary not just across age and race but also from community to community.

Among providers, awareness can be improved through provider-directed information regarding updated USPSTF and CMS guidelines and insurance coverage in the form of webinars, conferences, and accessible online resources with continued medical education (CME) credits.[15–18] This includes discussion and education surrounding the recent changes to reporting guidelines for LCS and how management differs between the previous and recently updated version.[19] These resources will help in the understanding of patient eligibility, in addition to management strategies for LCS recommendations and incidental findings.

The primary opportunity at the system level involves updating EMR systems to automatically identify eligible patients and inform both the provider and patient of their eligibility status, in addition

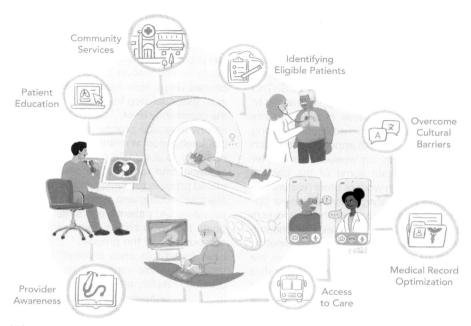

Fig. 1. Multifactorial barriers to lung cancer screening access exist at the individual, provider, and health system levels and impact many aspects of the patient's lung cancer screening care pathway. (*Courtesy of* Neha Udayakumar, MD, Boston, MA.)

to meeting future health care effectiveness data and information set quality measures related to LCS.[11] From a community perspective, bridging the gap between the bubble of health care and the community at large has been a challenge spanning a number of public health issues that have been exacerbated during the COVID-19 pandemic. Holding forums and informational sessions with community leaders and the general public may offer high-quality information to understand barriers related to access and stigma and to inform the development of community-based informational materials and programs aimed to increase LCS uptake.

LUNG CANCER SCREENING OPPORTUNITIES AND PARTICIPATION
Barriers

At the individual level, there are limited opportunities to provide or subsequently update one's smoking history, which is the linchpin in LCS eligibility (see **Fig. 1**). In addition, there may be cost concerns related to initial LCS examinations and subsequent recommended follow-up examinations and procedures in the event of a positive study or for evaluation of incidental findings.[10,19] Furthermore, a complex combination of factors, including managing competing life priorities, such as time off from work, navigating a fragmented health system, and stigma and anxiety related to annual screening and the potential of

an LC diagnosis are some of the factors that may prevent patients from enrolling in LCS.[11,20]

Among providers, it can be challenging to appropriately identify patients if their smoking history is incomplete or lacking in the opportunity to conduct shared decision-making and discuss LCS and any questions that may arise.[11,20] Furthermore, the lack of assistance in following up on incidental findings, and positive scans offer a barrier to implementation. Finally, the lack of access to accredited LCS centers within their system or without an optimized referral and follow-up process in an ever-expanding and complex health care system may create additional barriers to enrolling patients in LCS.

At the community and system level, some barriers include clear communication of services derived from LCS covered by payors, integrating telehealth services under the new CMS guidelines, and expanding broadband Internet access for communities. The lack of accredited radiology practices and centers to perform and interpret LCS examinations, decreased access to mobile LCS units among rural communities, and lack of an automated reminder and follow-up process are additional system-level barriers to meet patients where they and offer coordinated LCS care.[11,20,21]

Facilitators and Opportunities

At the individual level, opportunities for LCS include providing increased access to primary care services to disclose their smoking history, such as capturing the information through other health encounters or other nontraditional health care encounters such as health fares or pharmacies.[22] Facilitating care co-ordination and assisting in transportation challenges can also help increase opportunities for LCS. This could include grouping medical appointments to limit the number of times these outside barriers must be overcome.[23,24] In addition, offering increased flexibility in medical appointments, such as off-hour appointments on weekends and after work hours, can eliminate some of the barriers centered on time off from work or other responsibil-ities as caregivers. Creating comprehensive ap-pointments that include community health workers and patient navigators can help alleviate concerns centered on potential costs, assist in coordinating required follow-up appointments and improve the patient–provider relationship in a collaborative sense.[25] Finally, identifying concerns around stigma and radiation exposure, the American College of Radiology Lung Cancer Roundtable has launched a campaign with education efforts centered on these two barriers.[26–28]

From a provider perspective, linking LCS to con-versations and efforts surrounding tobacco cessa-tion and early cancer detection can be augmented by training around shared decision-making en-counters and the additional benefits of LCS in providing other clinically relevant health informa-tion, such as emphysema and coronary artery disease.[29,30] Other facilitators include increased collaboration with radiology practices' patient nav-igators to help manage both positive studies and incidental findings.[31] This removes some of the anxiety potentially centered on managing these re-sults while assisting patients in overcoming some of the barriers and allowing patients and referring providers to focus on smoking cessation and the global health trajectory of LCS.[32–34]

At the community and system level, policies combining updated USPSTF guidelines and social risk factors impacting the surrounding community can promote equity in LCS uptake.[7,11,13] Increasing available information about local accredited LCS centers via multiple mediums as well as languages is an essential step to disseminating information at the community level.[11] Optimization of the EMR via natural language processing and embedded artifi-cial intelligence algorithms offer an enormous op-portunity to automate much of the LCS selection, ordering, and reminder process. Having an auto-mated process to identify eligible patients, appoint-ment scheduling and reminder processes for both providers and patients, and streamlining the appro-priate follow-up orders could reduce some of the arduousness of the process.[11,35] Previous studies have found that once enrolled, underrepresented racial and ethnic minorities, as well as those who currently smoke, are less likely to remain enrolled in LCS. Furthermore, patients who continue to smoke while in LCS benefit from an integrated smoking cessation program that increases LCS participation and smoking cessation.[22,36] Last, a system-wide approach to coordinating with pa-tients who receive abnormal LCS results, either related to LC or an incidental finding, will benefit from a coordinated, patient-centered multidisci-plinary approach for managing possible LCs or other incidental findings.[37–39]

THE ROLE OF HUMANOMICS IN LUNG CANCER SCREENING AND FUTURE CONSIDERATIONS

Many of the multilevel barriers and opportunities directly impact the individual level. However, to this point, we have failed to systematically quantify the impact that structural discrimination and racism have at the biological level (**Fig. 2**). Recent studies

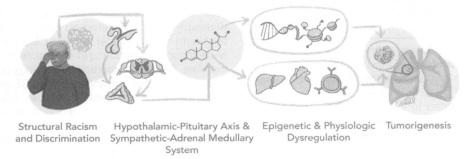

Structural Racism and Discrimination | Hypothalamic-Pituitary Axis & Sympathetic-Adrenal Medullary System | Epigenetic & Physiologic Dysregulation | Tumorigenesis

Fig. 2. In the model of humanomics, structural racism and discrimination (SRD) leads to increased allostatic load and activation of the hypothalamic–pituitary axis (HPA) and the sympathetic-adrenal medullary (SAM) system. In addition, increased activation of inflammatory markers and stress hormones, such as cortisol, alters the regula-tion of epigenetic, metabolic, cardiovascular, and immunological functions, which can promote tumorigenesis. (*Courtesy of* Neha Udayakumar, MD, Boston, MA.)

Table 1
Summary of multilevel barriers and facilitators to lung cancer screening

Levels	LCS Barriers and Facilitators	
	Awareness	**Opportunities and Participation**
Individual	Barriers: • Unawareness of LCS as screening tool, new USPSTF and CMS recommendations, and health insurance coverage • Uncertainty about available LCS programs • Lack of culturally appropriate information available at recommended health literacy levels Facilitators: • Creating educational content about LCS importance • Providing locations of nearby LCS centers • Providing culturally tailored education to fit the needs and capacities of diverse populations at an appropriate health literacy level	Barriers: • Undocumented smoking history • Health insurance coverage and costs unfamiliarity • Challenges understanding and following up LCS results • Conflicting personal and health schedules • Anxiety and stigma about LC diagnosis and radiation exposure Facilitators: • Providing accurate smoking history through educational campaigns or questionnaires during regular appointments • Providing same-day screening appointments at the time of other medical appointments • Appointments during weekends and evenings, providing transportation or mobile LCS units • Campaign with efforts in decreasing stigma associated with LC diagnosis and educating about alleviating radiation concerns • Increasing access to LCS clinics that offer an integrated approach to LCS in collaboration with primary care providers
Provider	Barriers: • Unfamiliarity with new USPSTF and CMS eligibility criteria • Unfamiliarity with insurance coverage and costs associated with LCS • Concerns related to the management of LCS and other incidental findings • Concern or skepticism about the clinical trial results Facilitators: • Providing provider, or clinic, specific educational material that offer CME credits • Providing educational webinars and institutional online resources for LCS	Barriers: • Difficulty identifying patients who meet eligibility criteria and understanding the influence of comorbidities • Inconsistent documented smoking history • Decreased access to multilingual decision aids • Reduced availability of LCS centers that do not offer a streamlined referral and follow-up process where patients can be referred to. • Lack of public transportation access to get to appointments Facilitators: • Training on shared decision-making encounters to gain further knowledge about tobacco cessation and benefits of LCS • EMR systems that assist in identifying eligible patients • Providing multilingual decision aids and providing tools to manage patient's emotions

(continued on next page)

Table 1
(*continued*)

Levels	LCS Barriers and Facilitators	
	Awareness	**Opportunities and Participation**
		• LCS radiology programs collaborating with primary care providers and community organizations by offering LCS, smoking cessation service and screening for other cancers
System/community	**Barriers:** • Institutional LCS information not tailored for the surrounding community's culture or language • EMR not optimized to notify providers of eligible patients	**Barriers:** • Barriers to telemedicine for conducting shared decision-making including decreased broadband Internet access in the community • Lack of health insurance coverage for LCS under new guidelines • EMR-based LCS appointment reminders not available in multiple languages or only through patient portals • Decreased availability of system-based dashboards that will alert about adherence to follow-up of abnormal LCS examinations
	Facilitators: • Creating EMR system-based alerts for LCS-eligible patients, with automated referral tools, and lists of certified LCS centers • Online Web site informational content that provides details to LCS programs with content tailored for the community at recommended health literacy level	**Facilitators:** • Increase efforts in providing community broadband Internet access and providing digital patient navigators to assist with patient portal enrollment • Increasing access to information about local accredited LCS centers • Optimizing EMR to identify population health level data of eligible patients under new guidelines • EMR-based LCS appointment reminders available in multiple languages and through additional services, such as text messaging • Updating population health dashboards alerts of eligible patients for LCS under the new guidelines to create system-based alerts

and models suggest that the mere aspect of living in an inequitable society dealing with systemic racism, overt hostility, and heightened vigilance leads to an increased level of baseline stress.[40] One model for discussing this increased stress is the allostatic load theory which describes increased activation of the hypothalamic–pituitary–adrenal axis due to exposure to societal pressures and negative SDoH.[8] Furthermore, the National Institute on Minority and Health Disparities has introduced a construct for considering the relationship between the general social environment and individual risk modifiers.[8,41] Therefore, to achieve the optimal goal of driving health equity through precision medicine, it is paramount to gain an in-depth understanding of how these social factors directly influence cancer outcomes through the biological effects of these social factors. This is where the role of social genomics and humanomics comes from, exploring how the psychological impact of negative societal factors impacts biological processes, including physiologic dysfunction and genomic changes.

We hypothesize that chronic psychosocial stress, such as that experienced due to structural racism and discrimination (SRD), leads to activation of the hypothalamic–pituitary axis and the sympathetic-adrenal medullary system and an increase in circulating inflammatory markers and stress hormones. Inflammation may directly mediate physiologic dysfunction in the cardiovascular (CVD), metabolic and immune systems, as well as contribute to reversible and irreversible changes in gene expression. Cumulatively, physiologic dysregulation and abnormal gene expression are hypothesized to lead to LC formation (see **Fig. 2**).

In breast cancer, one possible connection between stress-related gene expression and cancer is through the Conserved Transcriptional Response to Adversity (CTRA) RNA transcriptome. Described as early as 2007, this transcriptome expression is composed of pro-inflammatory genes (eg, interleukin [IL]1B, IL6, IL8, cyclooxygenase-2 [COX2], and tumor necrosis factor [TNF]) and antiviral genes. The increase in inflammatory gene expression and decrease in antiviral gene expression have been shown in this transcriptome in the setting of extended periods of adverse environmental conditions.[42,43] Patients with increased allostatic load may have increased CTRA expression as a possible link from societal factors to genetic modifications, although this requires dedicated evaluation. These links have been further studied in relation to specific outcomes related to cancers. For example, African ancestry, increased CTRA expression, and elevated IL6 expression have been linked to higher morbidity and mortality among Black patients with breast cancer.[44–48] Furthermore, direct CTRA expression in breast tumors has been associated with lower socioeconomic status and increased social isolation, offering an additional link between societal stressors and tumor development.[49–51] There is active work evaluating CTRA as a reversible marker for breast cancer risk.

The data on SRD-induced alteration in physiologic and genomic expression in the LC continuum are lacking. However, given the existing disparate outcomes among racial and ethnic minority patients and those with lower socioeconomic status markers, it is reasonable to suspect SRD indices have similar effects in LC that may explain gaps in LC outcomes among these high-priority populations. There is potential for CTRA and other physiologic or genomic markers to serve as precision risk markers in LC, mainly when applied to imaging-based screening. Further, future research can focus on the effects of social genomics, that is, gene expression related to societal exposures, on the appearance of disease on imaging (radiomics) to create a field of socioradiogenomic research. Furthermore, increased awareness and information about the possible links between societal stressors and individual genetics will likely offer new avenues to bridge existing and emerging disparities in LC outcomes effectively.

SUMMARY

To advance health equity in the LC care continuum through early detection, it is critical to do an in-depth evaluation of multilevel barriers to LCS and promote the creation of a multipronged foster LCS uptake among all eligible patients across different patient populations (**Table 1**). This includes further exploration into the role that systemic injustices and discrimination have on individuals and the specific genetics related to metaplasia and eventual LC formation. In a medical environment that is ever progressing toward personalized medicine, this is the next frontier. As radiologists, it is imperative that we take an active role in developing these strategies as well as implementing and participating in them as available.

CLINICS CARE POINTS

- Lung cancer screening (LCS) offers a unique opportunity to decrease existing lung cancer disparities among those communities disproportionately bearing the burden of increased morbidity and mortality from lung cancer.

- Understanding the intersection of societal structures and individual experiences through a humanomics model is crucial in our efforts to reduce disparities lung cancer mortality by increasing access to lung cancer screening.

- To advance health equity lung cancer care continuum, it is critical to do an in-depth evaluation of multilevel barriers to LCS that includes further exploration into the role that systemic discrimination have on genetics related to metaplasia and eventual lung cancer formation. This will inform the development of multipronged sustainable programs to enhance early detection with LCS and improve lung cancer outcomes for all.

DISCLOSURES

E.J. Flores reports grant funding from the National Cancer Institute, United States 1K08CA270430-01A1 related to the preparation of this article. Ruth Carlos reports salary support from the ACR as JACR Editor-in-Chief. Other authors have no commercial or financial conflicts of interest or funding sources related to the material herein.

REFERENCES

1. Siefel R, Miller K, Fuchs H, Jemal A. Cancer statistics, 2022 - Siegel - Wiley Online Library. ACS Journals. Available at: https://acsjournals.onlinelibrary.wiley.com/doi/10.3322/caac.21708. Published January 12, 2022.

2. Febbo J, Little B, Fischl-Lanzoni N, et al. Analysis of out-of-pocket cost of lung cancer screening for uninsured patients among ACR accredited imaging centers. J Am Coll Radiol 2020;17(9):1108–15.

3. Wang GX, Pizzi BT, Miles RC, et al. Implementation and utilization of a "pink card" walk-in screening mammography program integrated with physician visits. J Am Coll Radiol 2020;17(12):1602–8.

4. Doubeni CA, Simon M, Krist AH. Addressing systemic racism through clinical preventive service recommendations from the US preventive services task force. JAMA 2021;325(7):627–8.

5. Van Haren RM, Delman AM, Turner KM, et al. Impact of the COVID-19 pandemic on lung cancer screening program and subsequent lung cancer. J Am Coll Surg 2021;232(4):600–5.

6. US Preventive Services Task Force. Final recommendation statement: lung cancer: screening. Available at: https://www.uspreventiveservicestaskforce.org/uspstf/recommendation/lung-cancerscreening. Accessed March 9, 2021.

7. Cancer moonshot. The White House. Available at: https://www.whitehouse.gov/cancermoonshot/. Published August 9, 2022. Accessed March 25, 2023.

8. McEwen BS. Stress, adaptation, and disease. Allostasis and allostatic load. Ann N Y Acad Sci 1998; 840:33–44.

9. Ford JG, Howerton MW, Lai GY, et al. Barriers to recruiting underrepresented populations to cancer clinical trials: a systematic review. Cancer 2008; 112(2):228–42.

10. Trauth JM, Jernigan JC, Siminoff LA, et al. Factors affecting older African American women's decisions to join the PLCO Cancer Screening Trial. J Clin Oncol 2005;23:8730–8.

11. Wang G.X., Baggett T.P., Pandharipande P.V., et al., Barriers to Lung Cancer Screening Engagement from the Patient and Provider Perspective. Radiology, 290 (2), 2019, 278-287.

12. Wang GX, Neil JM, Fintelmann FJ, et al. Guideline discordant lung cancer screening: Emerging demand and provider indications. J Am Coll Radiol 2021;18:395–405.

13. Coughlin JM, Zang Y, Terranella S, et al. Understanding barriers to lung cancer screening in primary care. J Thorac Dis 2020;12(5):2536–44.

14. Gagne SM, Fintelmann FJ, Flores EJ, et al. Evaluation of the Informational Content and Readability of US Lung Cancer Screening Program Websites. JAMA Netw Open 2020;3(1):e1920431.

15. Lung National Training Network Internet. LuCa National Training Network. cited 2021Oct7. Available at: https://lucatraining.org/. Accessed March 1, 2023.

16. Jessup DL, Glover lv M, Daye D, et al. Implementation of digital awareness strategies to engage patients and providers in a lung cancer screening program: retrospective study. J Med Internet Res 2018;20(2):e52.

17. Lung Cancer Screening Resources Internet. American College of Radiology. cited 2021Oct7. Available at: https://www.acr.org/Clinical-Resources/Lung-Cancer-Screening-Resources. Accessed March 1, 2023.

18. Lung Rads Internet. Lung Rads | American College of Radiology. cited 2021Oct7. Available at: https://www.acr.org/Clinical-Resources/Reporting-and-Data-Systems/Lung-Rads. Accessed March 1, 2023.

19. National Lung Cancer Roundtable Lung Cancer Screening Webinar Series Internet. ACR Webinar. cited 2021Oct8. Available at: https://pages.acr.org/2021-NLCRT-Webinar-Series.html. Accessed March 1, 2023.

20. Lung Rads. Lung Rads | American College of Radiology. Available at: https://www.acr.org/Clinical-Resources/Reporting-and-Data-Systems/Lung-Rads. Accessed March 1, 2023.

21. Flores EJ, Irwin KE, Park ER, et al. Increasing lung screening in the Latino community. J Am Coll Radiol 2021;18(5):633–6.

22. Barbosa E Jr, Yang R, Hershman M. Real-world lung cancer CT screening performance, smoking behavior, and adherence to recommendations: lung-rads category and smoking status predict adherence. Am J Roentgenol 2021;216(4):919–26.

23. Cardarelli R, Roper KL, Cardarelli K, et al. Identifying community perspectives for a lung cancer screening awareness campaign in Appalachia Kentucky: The Terminate Lung Cancer (TLC) study. J Cancer Educ 2015;32(1):125–34.

24. Bieniasz ME, Underwood D, Bailey J, et al. Women's feedback on a chemopreventive trial for cervical dysplasia. Appl Nurs Res 2003;16(1):22–8.

25. Percac-Lima S, Ashburner J, Zai A, et al. Patient navigation for comprehensive cancer screening in high-risk patients using a population-based health information technology system: a randomized clinical trial. JAMA Intern Med 2016;176(7):930–7.

26. 'I've never been treated so well': Sameday cancer screening program helps reduce barriers Internet. Healio. cited 2021Sep29. Available at: https://www.healio.com/news/hematologyoncology/20210907/ive-never-been-treated-so-well-sameday-cancer-screening-program-helpsreduce-barriers29. Accessed March 1, 2023. Financial Assistance.

27. Lung cancer screening implementation guide Internet. American Thoracic Society. cited 2021Sep29.

Available at: https://www.lungcancerscreeningguide. org/. Accessed March 1, 2023.

28. Feldman J., Faris N.R., Warren G., Ending stigma in lung cancer: the IASLC participates in a collaborative summit held by the national lung cancer roundtable, *IASLC*, 2, 2020, 7-15. Available at: https://www.iaslc.org/iaslc-news/ilcn/ending-stigma-lung-cancer-iaslc-participatescollaborative-summit-held-national.

29. Christiani DC. Radiation risk from lung cancer screening. Chest 2014;145(3):439–40.

30. Fan L, Fan K. Lung cancer screening CT-based coronary artery calcification in predicting cardiovascular events: A systematic review and meta-analysis. Medicine (Baltim) 2018;97(20):e10461.

31. Hatabu H, Hunninghake GM, Richeldi L, et al. Interstitial lung abnormalities detected incidentally on CT: a Position Paper from the Fleischner Society. Lancet Respir Med 2020;8(7):726–37.

32. Module 3: Healthcare Team Internet. Community Health Workers and Patient Navigators. cited 2021Oct7. Available at: https://www.patient navigatortraining.org/healthcare_system/module3/ 8_community_health_workers_patient_navigators. htm. Accessed March 1, 2023.

33. Okpala P. Increasing access to primary health care through distributed leadership. Int J Healthc Manag 2021;14(3):914–9.

34. Joseph AM, Rothman AJ, Almirall D, et al. Lung cancer screening and smoking cessation clinical trials. SCALE (Smoking Cessation within the Context of Lung Cancer Screening) Collaboration. Am J Respir Crit Care Med 2018;197(2):172–82.

35. Headrick JR Jr, Morin O, Miller AD, et al. Mobile lung screening: should we all get on the bus? Ann Thorac Surg 2020;110(4):1147–52.

36. Hirsch EA, New ML, Brown SP, et al. Patient reminders and longitudinal adherence to lung cancer screening in an academic setting. Annals of the American Thoracic Society 2019;16(10):1329–32.

37. Lococo F, Cardillo G, Veronesi G. Does a lung cancer screening program promote smoking cessation? Thorax 2017;72(10):870–1.

38. Pulmonary nodule clinic Internet. Massachusetts General Hospital. cited 2021Oct7. Available at: https:// www.massgeneral.org/cancer-center/treatments-and-services/pulmonary-nodule-clinic. Accessed March 1, 2023.

39. Lung Screening Clinic Internet. MD Anderson Cancer Center. cited 2021Oct7. Available at: https://www. mdanderson.org/patients-family/diagnosis-treatment/ care-centers-clinics/cancerprevention-center/lung-screening-clinic.html. Accessed March 1, 2023.

40. ACR Designated lung cancer screening center Internet. Lung Cancer Screening Center. cited 2021Oct8. Available at: https://www.acraccreditation. org/lung-cancer-screeningcenter. Accessed March 1, 2023.

41. Agurs-Collins T, Persky S, Paskett ED, et al. Designing and assessing multilevel interventions to improve minority health and reduce health disparities. Am J Publ Health 2019;109:S86–93.

42. Alvidrez J, Castille D, Laude-Sharp M, et al. The National Institute on Minority Health and Health Disparities research framework. Am J Publ Health 2019; 109:S16–20.

43. Cole SW, Hawkley LC, Arevalo JM, et al. Social regulation of gene expression in human leukocytes. Genome Biol 2007;8:1–13.

44. Cole SW. Human social genomics. PLoS Genet 2014;10:e1004601.

45. Schneider BP, Shen F, Jiang G, et al. Impact of genetic ancestry on outcomes in ECOG-ACRIN-E5103. JCO Precis Oncol 2017. https://doi.org/10. 1200/PO.17.00059.

46. Bachelot T, Ray-Coquard I, Menetrier-Caux C, et al. Prognostic value of serum levels of interleukin 6 and of serum and plasma levels of vascular endothelial growth factor in hormone-refractory metastatic breast cancer patients. Br J Cancer 2003;88: 1721–6.

47. Obeng-Gyasi S, O'Neill AM, Miller K, et al. Social determinants of health, genetic ancestry, and mortality in ECOG-ACRIN E5103. J Clin Oncol 2021;39 (15_ suppl; abstr 6527).

48. Sparano JA, O'Neill AM, Graham N, et al. Inflammatory cytokines and distant recurrence in HER2-negative early breast cancer in the ECOG-ACRIN 5103 trial. J Clin Oncol 2021;39 (15_suppl; abstr 520).

49. Akinyemiju T, Wilson LE, Deveaux A, et al. Association of allostatic load with all-cause and cancer mortality by race and body mass index in the REGARDS cohort. Cancers 2020;12:1695.

50. Bower JE, Shiao SL, Sullivan P, et al. Prometastatic molecular profiles in breast tumors from socially isolated women. JNCI Cancer Spectr 2018;2:pky029.

51. Carlos R., Obeng-Gyasi S., Cole S., et al., Linking structural racism and discrimination and breast cancer outcomes: a social genomics approach, *J Clin Oncol*, 40 (13), 2022, 1407-1413. Available at: https://pubmed.ncbi.nlm.nih.gov/35108027/.

Lung Cancer Screening
The European Perspective

Piergiorgio Muriana, MD[a], Francesca Rossetti, MD[a], Pierluigi Novellis, MD[a], Giulia Veronesi, MD[a,b],*

KEYWORDS

- Lung cancer • Screening • European • Low-dose CT • Prevention • Mortality • Biomarker
- Artificial intelligence

KEY POINTS

- Large randomized trials demonstrated that screening with low-dose computed tomography (CT) reduces mortality from lung cancer in active and former smokers.
- Primary prevention with smoking cessation counseling improves cost-effectiveness of lung cancer screening.
- Candidates should be selected according to estimation of lung cancer development risk.
- Volumetric low-dose CT and fludeoxyglucose -PET can limit false positive rate and unnecessary invasive procedures.
- Circulating biomarkers assessment and computer-assisted diagnosis software may further improve the accuracy and cost-effectiveness of lung cancer screening.

INTRODUCTION

Lung cancer is still a major responsible for oncological morbidity and mortality worldwide. According to the analysis of GLOBOCAN 2020 database, in 2020 over 2 million people developed lung cancer, representing 11.4% of all cases of tumors, and almost 1.8 million people died of the disease.[1] In the 27 member countries of the European Union (EU) it has been estimated that in 2023 lung cancer will be the first cause of tumor death in males (over 159,000 new deaths), and the second one in the female sex following breast cancer (83,553 deaths).[2]

Variations in trends of lung cancer incidence and mortality are closely related to tobacco consumption. The efforts in primary prevention promoting smoking cessation led to a reduction of all-sites cancer rates compared to 35 years ago. However, this is not completely true for lung cancer: although there has been a reduction in lung cancer mortality in men both in the United Kingdom and the EU countries since 1970 and 1985, respectively, unfavorable rates are still observed among women in the most advanced age groups. In fact, lung cancer incidence is currently rising in highly populated European nations such as France, Italy, and Spain. Moreover, a considerable proportion of new lung cancer cases are related to factors other than smoking, such as air pollution, asbestos, and radon exposure.[3]

To aim to an effective reduction of lung cancer incidence, it is necessary to establish measures at different levels, that is, controlling environmental and occupational pollution, applying tobacco restriction policies, settling primary prevention programs to increase social awareness of smoking-related harms, and favoring secondary prevention with lung cancer screening (LCS) programs in selected high-risk population.

LUNG CANCER SURVIVAL AND THE IMPACT OF LUNG CANCER SCREENING PROGRAMS

The prognosis of patients affected by lung cancer is poor, with 5-year overall survival (OS) ranging from 10% to 20%. This is strictly dependent on

[a] Department of Thoracic Surgery, San Raffaele Scientific Institute, Via Olgettina 60, Milan 20132, Italy;
[b] School of Medicine and Surgery, Vita-Salute San Raffaele University, Via Olgettina 48, Milan 20132, Italy
* Corresponding author. Department of Thoracic Surgery, San Raffaele Scientific Institute, Via Olgettina, 60, Milan 20132, Italy.
E-mail address: veronesi.giulia@hsr.it

Thorac Surg Clin 33 (2023) 375–383
https://doi.org/10.1016/j.thorsurg.2023.04.017
1547-4127/23/© 2023 Elsevier Inc. All rights reserved.

disease stage at diagnosis[4]: in fact, 5Y-OS ranges from about 60% in case of localized tumor, to 34% in patients with locoregional disease, and to only 7% in case of metastatic disease.[5,6]

Certainly, lack of signs and symptoms in early-stage lung cancer is the main cause of delayed diagnosis, with nearly 70% of stage I non-small cell lung cancer (NSCLC) patients being asymptomatic; when present, occurrence of each single symptom is aspecific.[7] As a result, 44% of all patients have distant metastases at diagnosis, whereas only 26% have early-stage cancers.[5]

By contrast, in the International Early Lung Cancer Action Project (I-ELCAP), an LCS program on over 31,000 high-risk subjects who underwent annual spiral computed tomography (CT) between 1993 and 2005, 85% of patients with lung cancer were diagnosed with clinical stage I tumor. Within this group, the 10-year OS reached 88%, and resulted even better (92%) among the patients treated with radical surgical resection.[8]

More recently, in a randomized controlled trial (RCT) performed in the United States on 53,454 high-risk individuals—the National Lung Screening Trial (NLST), subjects screened with 3 annual rounds of low-radiation-dose CT (LDCT) showed 20% reduction in lung cancer mortality compared to those enrolled in a homogeneous chest X-ray (CXR) group ($P = 0.004$).[9] Also, the rate of death from any cause was significantly lowered in the LDCT group by 6.7% ($P = 0.02$).

The NLST study was the first large RCT to demonstrate the efficacy of LCS in preventing mortality from lung cancer in high-risk subjects. Of note, these effects on mortality were probably even underestimated because of the short screening window (3 years) with no additional rounds. The trial did not include a primary prevention program.

Based on the outcomes of NLST, LDCT has become the gold standard technique in LCS in high-risk smokers.[10] Meanwhile, other RCTs and single-arm LCS studies have been designed in Europe and around the world.[11–15]

POPULATION AT RISK AND POTENTIAL CANDIDATES TO LUNG CANCER SCREENING

One the major issues encountered by NLST was to obtain an appropriate balance between inclusion criteria, a protocol design able to minimize false positives (FP), and costs related to a large-scale LCS. At that time, the authors noted that only 7 million over 94 million current and former smokers in the United States met inclusion criteria established by the trial, leaving behind a significant number of people developing lung cancer because of risk factors other than active smoking.[9]

According to a secondary analysis of the Continuous Observation of Smoking Subjects (COSMOS) study,[13] it was estimated that about 12.2% of over 17 million current and former smokers in Italy were at risk of developing lung cancer based on population data obtained in 2017 and application of US Preventive Services Task Force (USPSTF) selection criteria.[16]

Recently, in a budget analysis for the implementation of LCS in Europe, the establishment of national LCS programs in 28 European countries could prevent more than 18,000 deaths for lung cancer over 21 million high-risk subjects at a sustainable cost of about 50,000 euros/per-person-saved.[17]

THE EUROPEAN EXPERIENCE ON LUNG CANCER SCREENING: RANDOMIZED AND OBSERVATIONAL STUDIES

Several LCS studies are currently in progress across Europe, both with RCT and single-arm observational design.[18] Study design, inclusion criteria, and major results are listed in **Table 1**.

The Detection and Screening of Early Lung Cancer by Imaging Technology and Molecular Essays Study

The Detection and Screening of Early Lung Cancer by Imaging Technology and Molecular Essays (DANTE) trial was a prospective RCT initiated in 2001. The primary aim of the study was to evaluate the impact of LDCT screening on lung cancer mortality as compared to repeated clinical assessments.

The first analysis of the DANTE study after 3 years of follow-up failed to demonstrate a significant benefit of LDCT screening: although more lung cancers overall (4.7% vs. 2.8%, $P = 0.016$) and more early-stage tumors (2.6% vs. 1.0%, $P = 0.004$) were diagnosed in the screened group, no difference in overall and cancer-specific mortality ($P = 0.83$ and $P = 0.84$) was demonstrated.[11] A later review of the study confirmed these results after a median follow-up of 8 years.[19]

The Multicentric Italian Lung Detection Study and the Results of Pooled Analysis with Detection and Screening of Early Lung Cancer by Imaging Technology and Molecular Essays Trial

In 2012, Pastorino and colleagues[12] presented the 5-year follow-up results of the Multicentric Italian Lung Detection (MILD) study. Participants were randomized in 3 cohorts: no screening, annual LDCT, and biennial LDCT, with all being enrolled

Table 1
Details and results of previous lung cancer screening trials with low-dose computed tomography

Trial ID, Study Design, Country, Recruitment Period	Inclusion Criteria (Age, Smoking Pack/Year, Abstinence Years, %Males)	N Screening Group	N Control Group	%Adherence	Screening Rounds, Frequency	Volumetric Evaluation	Recall Threshold	%Recall Rate	Follow-up (Median, Years)	%False Positive	%Stage I Lung Cancer	Primary Outcome
I-ELCAP,[8] single-arm, multinational, 1993–2005	≥40, no limits, passive smokers and occupational exposure included	31,567	None	87	NR, annual	No	D ≥ 5 mm; none at follow-up	13 at baseline, 5 at follow-up	NR	NR	85	10Y-OS = 88% in early stage LDCT detected tumors undergoing surgery
NLST,[9] RCT, USA, 2002–2004	55–74, ≥30, ≤15, 59	26,722	26,732 (CXR)	95	3, annual	No	D ≥ 4 mm	24.2	12.3	23.3	50	20% lung cancer mortality reduction with LDCT[a]
DANTE,[11,19] RCT, Italy, 2001–2006	60–74, ≥20, <10, 100	1264	1186	94	5, annual	No	None	28	8.4	17.7[b]	64	No lung cancer mortality advantage with LDCT
MILD,[12,21] RCT, Italy, 2005–2011	49–75, ≥20, <10, 66	2376 (1190 annual, 1186 biennial)	1723	96 (annual), 95 (biennial)	4–7, (annual or biennial)	Yes	D ≥ 5 mm, V ≥ 60 mL	15 (annual), 14 (biennial)	6.2	4.6[b]	50	39% lung cancer mortality reduction with LDCT on prolonged follow-up[a]
ITALUNG,[14] RCT, Italy, 2004–2006	55–69, ≥20, ≤10, 64	1613	1593	81	4, annual	No	D ≥ 5 mm	52.7	9.3	NR	36	30% lung cancer mortality reduction with LDCT
COSMOS,[13,26] single-arm, Italy, 2004–2005	≥50, ≥20, ≤10, 66	5203	None	79	5, annual	Yes	D > 5 mm, VDT ≤400 d	6.4	NR	14[b]	78	A structured protocol LCS enhance the identification of high rate of curable lung cancer with negligible harm
NELSON,[15] RCT, Netherlands/Belgium, 2003–2006	50–75, ≥15 cig/d for 25 y or ≥10 cig for 30 y, ≤10, 84	6583	6612	90	4, at 1-2-2.5 y after baseline	Yes	D ≥ 5 mm, V ≥ 50 mL, VDT ≤600 d	20.4	8.2	1.2	59	24% lung cancer mortality reduction with LDCT (males)[a]

Abbreviations: D, diameter; NR, not reported; V, volume.
[a] Statistical significant.
[b] Received surgery.

in a smoking cessation program as well. The rationale for biennial CT lies in the attempt to enhance the LCS economical sustainability and to reduce radiation exposure without negatively influencing the accuracy of lung cancer detection. Moreover, automated computer-assisted diagnosis (CAD) volumetric evaluation and fluorodeoxyglucose (FDG)-PET scan were systematically employed in the diagnostic work-up of suspicious lesions found at screening rounds. This resulted in a drop in invasive procedures for benign disease compared to previous experiences (9%).

Although the incidence of lung cancer was higher in the screened groups than in the control cohort ($P = 0.025$), both overall and lung cancer mortality did not differ among the 3 arms of the study ($P = 0.13$ and $P = 0.21$).

Still, an important outcome of the trial was the demonstration of equivalence of biennial and yearly LDCT rounds in the identification of stage I (70% vs. 62%, $P = 0.53$) and resectable disease (85% vs. 83%, $P = 0.57$).[12]

A pooled analysis of both MILD and DANTE database, including over 3600 LDCT screened persons and over 2900 nonscreened subjects with long-term follow-up (median 8.2 years), demonstrated nonsignificant 11% reduction in overall mortality and 17% reduction in cancer-specific mortality in the LDCT group. The authors noted that a reduction in cancer mortality was evident after 4 years of follow-up, suggesting that a significant reduction in mortality can be observed by extending the follow-up beyond 8 years.[20]

Actually, a further analysis aimed at evaluating long-term overall and lung cancer specific mortality in MILD study participants: although no significant difference was demonstrated in terms of overall mortality, cancer mortality risk was reduced to 1.7% in the study group compared with 2.5% of the control arm [hazard ratio (HR) = 0.61, $P = 0.02$] after 10 years of follow-up, confirming a major advantage of prolonged LCS.[21]

The Italian Lung Cancer Study

The Italian Lung Cancer (ITALUNG) screening trial randomized a screening group undergoing LDCT annually for 4 years, and a control group receiving standard care.

After a median follow-up of 9.3 years, even though this trial failed to prove the primary outcome statistically, the LDCT group showed 30% reduction in lung cancer specific mortality and 17% reduction in overall mortality ($P = 0.07$ and $P = 0.08$). Furthermore, the study group showed no overdiagnosis, being the number of encountered lung cancers similar to controls

[relative risk (RR) = 0.93]. On the other hand, more early-stage disease and surgically treatable cases were identified through active screening ($P < 0.001$ and $P = 0.003$).[14]

The Continuous Observation of Smoking Subjects Study

The COSMOS study was designed as a single-arm LCS trial enrolling in 1 year 5203 high-risk subjects and then following them up for 10 years with annual LDCT.

After the first 5 years of follow-up, lung cancer was diagnosed in 175 patients, 78% of whom presented as stage I disease. R0 resection was achieved in 87% of surgical cases with low morbidity. Minimally invasive robotic approach was adopted in 27.4% of patients. 5Y-OS of patients who underwent surgery was 78%.[13] This observational trial aimed at proving the feasibility of LCS in a real-world population based on the application of a structured protocol to limit FP occurrence requiring additional investigations, overdiagnosis, and possible screening-induced harms.

Several important results were obtained. First, the integration in the protocol of selective PET scan for the evaluation of larger nodules (>8 mm) or those progressively enlarging[22] allowed low recall (6.4% overall) and invasive procedure rates. Only 14% of patients undergoing surgical biopsy of suspicious lesions resulted benign. Volume-doubling time (VDT) was another important factor guiding clinicians in the diagnostic process. Patients with cancers appearing at follow-up and those with VDT less than 400 days (fast growing) showed a poorer prognosis than indolent tumors (VDT ≥600 days) due to higher rates of lung cancer specific mortality (9.2% vs. 4.1% vs. 0.9% per year).[23]

Differently from most other models focused on the selection of target population, a new lung cancer risk model to define an appropriate screening interval was delineated. This model employs epidemiologic (eg, age and smoking habits) and baseline CT information (presence of emphysema, eventual nodule characteristics, and others) to evaluate the annual risk of lung cancer development,[24] and it has recently been validated in a study in which subjects at low risk (<0.6%) were followed up with biennial LDCT, whereas those at high-risk were screened yearly. The 2 groups showed significantly different lung cancer/CT ratio (1/55 vs. 1/31, respectively), confirming that biennial follow-up is adequate for the LCS of low-risk subjects reducing costs and potential radiation-induced hazard.[25]

After 10-year follow-up, only one case of radiation-induced major cancers per 108 lung tumors detected was reported, which can be regarded as negligible considering the potential mortality reduction effect achievable by early treatment of pulmonary tumors identified by LCS. Moreover, it should be highlighted that radiation exposure may be reduced even more with future technological advancements of CT scanners, modulation of LDCT protocols, and application of tailored LCS intervals.[26]

The Dutch-Belgian Nederlands–Leuvens Longkanker Screenings Onderzoek Study

In 2020, the results of 10-year follow up of the large randomized Dutch-Belgian Nederlands–Leuvens Longkanker Screenings Onderzoek (NELSON) study were published.[15] This population-based trial has largely been advocated because of its strong statistical power to confirm at the European level the benefit on lung cancer mortality given by LCS in high-risk population as shown in the NLST.

Data on 13,195 male subjects were available for analysis, randomized 1:1 into a screening group undergoing baseline LDCT screening and subsequent follow-up with intervals of 1, 2, and 2.5 years, and a control, nonscreened group. Moreover, additional recruitment of female candidates resulted in a secondary analysis on 2594 women. Differently from the NLST study, CT-detected nodules were further analyzed by a semiautomated segmentation software with possible double reading by a specialized radiologist to determine nodule volume and VDT.

At the end of follow-up, bare lung cancer mortality ratio resulted significantly lower in the screening group than in controls for men (0.76, $P = 0.01$), with an even stronger efficacy in the small group of women (0.67). Regarding the primary analysis in the male population, overall incidence of tumors was higher in the study group (5.58 vs. 4.91 tumors/1000 person-year), with a higher proportion of early-stage disease diagnosis (58.6% vs. 13.5%). By contrast, metastatic disease resulted more frequent in the control group than in the screening cohort (45.7% vs. 9.4%). Another major outcome of this study was the evidence that the survival benefit of LCS in high-risk individuals lasted up to 11 years of follow-up.[15] Work-up harms (FP rate and recurrence to invasive tests) were limited and did not influence favorable outcomes.

In the accompanying editorial of the NELSON study,[27] Duffy and Field put attention on other important evidences from this trial, such as the efficacy of progressively longer screening intervals

with potential superiority of biennial follow-up on radiation-induced toxicity and cost benefit. As stated by these authors, "with the NELSON results, the efficacy of low-dose CT screening for lung cancer is confirmed. Our job is no longer to assess whether low-dose CT screening for lung cancer works: it does. Our job is to identify the target population in which it will be acceptable and cost-effective."

THE PROBLEM OF ENROLLMENT AND AN EXAMPLE OF EFFECTIVE COMMUNICATION: THE TARGETED LUNG HEALTH CHECK PROGRAM

Defining the most appropriate criteria is not the only challenge of LCS enrollment. Other factors of informative, logistic, and economic nature may influence poor adhesion, in particular in most disadvantaged social groups. Moreover, it is a common opinion that all smoking-related diseases may be perceived as self-induced, with the risk of community stigmatization, and subsequent lower recurrence to medical assistance.[28]

The Targeted Lung Health Check (THLC) program was an implementation LCS study initiated in the district of Manchester (UK) in 2016. Several strategies have been adopted to favor the adhesion socially frail subjects. First, the trial itself was identified with the generalist term of "lung health check" to enhance dissociation of the screening process from smoking habit considerations and lung cancer, therefore reducing the risk of negative perception. Second, recruitment was carried out close to shopping centers and other social facilities, and LDCTs were acquired by mobile scanners. These approaches led to an improvement in the participation of high-risk population with potential access problems to medical structures. Finally, they adopted a policy of continuative information of the process workflow, improving the perception of candidates of being active part of the study. This model allowed high rates of early-stage lung cancer detection (80.4%), curative resection (65%), and positive cost-effectiveness evaluation in low-income population compared to demographic data in the UK.[29,30]

THE EUROPEAN VIEW ON COST-EFFECTIVENESS ANALYSIS OF LUNG CANCER SCREENING

The proof of a favorable ratio between LCS costs and effectiveness on lung cancer morbidity and mortality reduction is one of the major issues affecting the implementation of national LCS programs. In literature, several studies evaluated the

CEA of many LCS programs under different points of view. What is evident is that a plethora of factors, both country-related (eg, national income, health system regimen) and LCS-related (eg, inclusion criteria, diagnostic work-up, management of findings, and others), have a strong influence on the assessment of positive CEA.

In most studies, CEA quantification is reported as incremental cost-effectiveness ratio (ICER), which is the difference in cost between LCS and no screening, divided by the difference in quality-adjusted life-year (QALY) gained. A previous analysis of the NLST database showed that ICER of LDCT screening would amount to 81,000$ per QALY. However, this result was considerably influenced by a number of variables, such as age, gender, smoking status, and individual lung cancer risk.[31]

CEA of LCS is highly variable across Europe; nevertheless, most studies conclude in favor of screening advantage under an economical aspect. An economical evaluation of THLC program estimated an ICER of about 10,000£/QALY, resulting well below the ideal threshold (20,000–30,000£) applied by the National Institute for Health and Excellence (NICE) for the proper allocation of NHS funds allocation.[30]

We recently published the CEA of the Italian COSMOS study, which showed an even more favorable ICER amounting to 3297€/QALY, considering real-world data evaluated by hospital records and new immunotherapy treatment for patients with locally-advanced or metastatic disease. Under the assumptions of this study, and after the estimation of people at risk, we demonstrated that costs of population screening are economically sustainable, requiring about 600 million euros to finance a 5-year LCS at the Italian national level.[16]

UPDATED RECOMMENDATIONS FOR LUNG CANCER SCREENING IN EUROPE

In the light of the results of trials in Europe and across the world, several scientific societies released specific indications addressing the application and implementation of LCS programs both at local, national, and international level.

Since guidelines on the management of early-stage lung cancer were released by the European Society of Medical Oncology (ESMO) in 2017 (before the NELSON trial results), the implementation of large-scale LCS by LDCT could not be recommended, waiting for confirmation of lung cancer mortality reduction as resulted in NLST.[32]

The European Society of Thoracic Surgeons (ESTS) suggested an active involvement of the European Commission to enhance public LCS programs, focusing on risk models application, the efficacy of biennial screening, the reduction of FP, and the improvement of minimally invasive treatment of positive cases. Smoking cessation projects were strongly recommended.[33]

In 2020, in the light of survival results of the largest RCTs, the European Society of Radiology (ESR) and the European Respiratory Society (ERS) agreed that it was high time to establish population-based organized pathways for lung cancer early detection in high-risk subjects, supported by European healthcare systems. In line with ESTS guidelines,[33] this document stressed the use of appropriate communication during recruitment, the utilization of risk-estimation models, the association of primary prevention to LCS, and the application of diagnostic algorithms including PET scan, volumetric analysis, and CAD to ensure high accuracy with low FP rate and beneficial cost-effectiveness balance.[28]

Following a systematic review of the literature, the recommendations of ESR/ERS were strengthened by the Initiative for European Lung Cancer Screening (IELS) expert group[34] underlining the added value of LDCT screening to improve the prevention and early treatment of other smoking-related diseases like cardiovascular diseases (through calcium score assessment on nongated LDCT), and pulmonary diseases like emphysema and chronic obstructive pulmonary disease (COPD).[34]

Finally, in 2022 the Science Advice for Policy by European Academies (SAPEA) consortium released an evidence review report aimed at improving cancer screening in Europe. Based on the proven LCS effect on lung cancer mortality in high-risk population with concurrent reasonably acceptable harm, LCS is now included between those recommended for implementation in Europe as population-based programs.[35]

Actually, the present situation of LCS in Europe is still heterogeneous. National trials are currently ongoing in Croatia, Poland, and Czech Republic, and are under evaluation in other countries.[18] In Italy, the Ministry of Health evaluates the implementation of a national pilot study aimed at reaching 7% of target population in 3 years.

FUTURE PERSPECTIVES: THE ROLE OF BIOMARKERS AND ARTIFICIAL INTELLIGENCE IN LUNG CANCER SCREENING

Striving for optimization of LCS by reducing related harms, better efficacy could be obtained by the inclusion of potentially reliable biomarkers in lung cancer risk assessment and differential diagnosis of lung nodules, and radiomic analysis through artificial intelligence (AI) systems to detect and characterize lesions.

Currently, even if there is still no validated set of biomarkers, interesting results were reported by analyses conducted on screen-eligible population. The Italian BioMILD study assessed the role of serum microRNA (miRNA) signature to evaluate lung cancer risk among participants and define tailored screening intervals. Risk stratification according to baseline negative LDCT and circulating miRNA assay allows the selection of LCS participants that can undergo triennial rounds because of low cancer probability and better survival. Therefore, if independent validation will be obtained, miRNA evaluation could have an important role in the diagnostic work-up of screening-diagnosed lesions.[36] Montani and colleagues[37] initially confirmed the potential diagnostic role of circulating miRNA signature, even if validation was not obtained in the second cohort of COSMOS study.

The ongoing Smokers health Multiple Actions (SMAC) program aims at implementing comprehensive early diagnosis of lung cancer and other smoking-related "big killers" like COPD and cardiovascular diseases. Individuals with 6-year lung cancer risk greater than 2% according to PLCOm2012 model[38] undergo baseline LDCT, blood collection, spirometry, and smoking cessation counseling. Suspicious lesions are evaluated through segmentation and volumetry to define the following work-up. The presence of emphysema and/or coronary calcification is evaluated to decide on the need for pneumologic and cardiologic consult. In case of negative LDCT, screening interval (annual/biennial) is calculated according to Maisonneuve risk model.[25] The assessment of multiple molecular biomarkers related to the target diseases is integrated: circulating tumor cells with genomic analysis, miRNA and PTX3 for lung cancer, IL-2 and IL-8 for COPD, miRNA for cardiovascular diseases. The primary aim of both primary prevention and serum biomarkers association with LDCT is to strengthen the program sensitivity and improve cost-effectiveness.

The role of AI in the field of LCS has been explored in a secondary analysis of the NELSON study. The performance of CAD was compared with radiologist double reading. CAD analysis showed higher sensitivity than double reading (96.7% vs. 78.1%), but a major drawback was related to occurrence of a significant rate of FP per examination (3.7 vs. 0.5). After exclusion of smaller volume nodules (<50 mL), a drop to 1.9 FP/examination and increase of positive predictive value were observed. Notably, 21.9% of lesions requiring further assessment were detected by CAD only.[39]

Certainly, the development of advanced deep-learning CAD systems, especially those based on convolutional neural networks technology, may further improve the performance of AI-assisted LCS.[40] It is reasonable that several advantages could be expected: better quality images enabling the introduction of ultra-LDCT; embedment of radiomic and biohumoral information; better lung cancer risk estimation leading to tailored screening protocols; and positive economic impact allowing the enhancement of programs in lower income countries.

In 2022, the French lung Cancer Screening using low-dose CT and Artificial intelligence for Detection (CASCADE) trial started the enrollment of 2400 asymptomatic women at risk to explore the greater benefit of LCS in the female gender. This modern prospective observational study has the primary goal to compare the accuracy of LDCT reading by a single AI-assisted radiologist trained in LCS with that of double reading. Additionally, AI reading alone performance will be evaluated as one of secondary outcomes.[41]

SUMMARY

Two large RCTs in the United States and in Europe have confirmed that LCS with LDCT decreases lung cancer mortality thanks to identification and early treatment of limited disease. As LCS-associated harm concern still exists, in particular related to test accuracy, to radiation-induced adverse effects, and to costs, an active involvement of European institutions has come to promote the development of public LCS programs, with multiple aims focused on quality control to reduce potential harm, the improvement of primary prevention, accessibility, and screening workflow.

CLINICS CARE POINTS

- In the recruitment process of LCS, a risk prediction model (as PLCOm2012) should be implemented to improve selection of target population;
- In the diagnostic algorithm of LCS, volumetric LDCT, FDG-PET for suspicious nodules, and eventual biopsy (transbronchial or CT-guided) should be included to allow a reduction of FP undergoing invasive surgical procedures;
- Multidisciplinary discussion of positive cases is recommended;
- Personalized screening intervals with biennal rounds for CT-negative participants allow us to reduce LCS harm due to cumulative radiation exposure and costs;

- Smoking cessation programs should be offered to all screening smokers to reduce smoking exposure and improve cost-effectiveness of LCS;
- Minimally invasive (robotic or VATS) surgery and sublobar resection should be offered to patients with early-stage lung cancer.

DISCLOSURE

Dr P. Muriana, Dr F. Rossetti, and Dr P. Novellis have no conflict of interest to declare. Prof. G. Veronesi received grants from Umberto Veronesi Foundation, Italy, Intuitive Surgical, United States, AIRC, Italy, Italian Ministry of Health, Italy and INAIL, Italy; she is a consultant for Ab Medica SpA, Medtronic, Astra Zeneca and Roche.

REFERENCES

1. Sung H, Ferlay J, Siegel RL, et al. Global Cancer Statistics 2020: GLOBOCAN Estimates of Incidence and Mortality Worldwide for 36 Cancers in 185 Countries. CA Cancer J Clin 2021;71(3):209–49.
2. Malvezzi M, Santucci C, Boffetta P, et al. European Cancer Mortality Predictions For The Year 2023 With Focus On Lung Cancer. Ann Oncol 2023; 34(4):410–9.
3. Turner MC, Andersen ZJ, Baccarelli A, et al. Outdoor air pollution and cancer: An overview of the current evidence and public health recommendations. CA Cancer J Clin 2020;70(6):460–79.
4. Allemani C, Matsuda T, Di Carlo V, et al. Global surveillance of trends in cancer survival 2000-14 (CONCORD-3): analysis of individual records for 37 513 025 patients diagnosed with one of 18 cancers from 322 population-based registries in 71 countries. Lancet 2018;391(10125):1023–75.
5. Siegel RL, Miller KD, Wagle NS, et al. Cancer statistics, 2023. CA Cancer J Clin 2023;73(1):17–48.
6. Goldstraw P, Chansky K, Crowley J, et al. The IASLC Lung Cancer Staging Project: Proposals for Revision of the TNM Stage Groupings in the Forthcoming (Eighth) Edition of the TNM Classification for Lung Cancer. J Thorac Oncol 2016;11(1):39–51.
7. Ruano-Raviña A, Provencio M, Calvo De Juan V, et al. Lung cancer symptoms at diagnosis: results of a nationwide registry study. ESMO Open 2020; 5(6):e001021.
8. International Early Lung Cancer Action Program Investigators, Henschke CI, Yankelevitz DF, et al. Survival of patients with stage I lung cancer detected on CT screening. N Engl J Med 2006;355(17):1763–71.
9. National Lung Screening Trial Research Team, Aberle DR, Adams AM, et al. Reduced lung-cancer mortality with low-dose computed tomographic screening. N Engl J Med 2011;365(5):395–409.
10. Krist AH, Davidson KW, Mangione CM, et al. Screening for Lung Cancer: US Preventive Services Task Force Recommendation Statement. JAMA 2021;325(10):962–70.
11. Infante M, Cavuto S, Lutman FR, et al. A randomized study of lung cancer screening with spiral computed tomography: three-year results from the DANTE trial. Am J Respir Crit Care Med 2009;180(5):445–53.
12. Pastorino U, Rossi M, Rosato V, et al. Annual or biennial CT screening versus observation in heavy smokers: 5-year results of the MILD trial. Eur J Cancer Prev 2012;21(3):308–15.
13. Veronesi G, Maisonneuve P, Spaggiari L, et al. Diagnostic performance of low-dose computed tomography screening for lung cancer over five years. J Thorac Oncol 2014;9(7):935–9.
14. Paci E, Puliti D, Lopes Pegna A, et al. Mortality, survival and incidence rates in the ITALUNG randomised lung cancer screening trial. Thorax 2017; 72(9):825–31.
15. de Koning HJ, van der Aalst CM, de Jong PA, et al. Reduced Lung-Cancer Mortality with Volume CT Screening in a Randomized Trial. N Engl J Med 2020;382(6):503–13.
16. Veronesi G, Navone N, Novellis P, et al. Favorable incremental cost-effectiveness ratio for lung cancer screening in Italy. Lung Cancer 2020;143:73–9.
17. Pan X, Dvortsin E, Aerts J, et al. P1.02-03 Budget Impact Analysis of Volume CT Lung Cancer Screening Based on NELSON Study Outcomes in Europe. J Thorac Oncol 2022;17(9):S99.
18. The Lung Cancer Policy Network. Interactive map of lung cancer screening. Available at: https://www.lungcancerpolicynetwork.com/interactive-map-of-lung-cancer-screening/. Accessed March 29, 2023.
19. Infante M, Cavuto S, Lutman FR, et al. Long-Term Follow-up Results of the DANTE Trial, a Randomized Study of Lung Cancer Screening with Spiral Computed Tomography. Am J Respir Crit Care Med 2015;191(10):1166–75.
20. Infante M, Sestini S, Galeone C, et al. Lung cancer screening with low-dose spiral computed tomography: evidence from a pooled analysis of two Italian randomized trials. Eur J Cancer Prev 2017;26(4):324–9.
21. Pastorino U, Silva M, Sestini S, et al. Prolonged lung cancer screening reduced 10-year mortality in the MILD trial: new confirmation of lung cancer screening efficacy. Ann Oncol 2019;30(7):1162–9.
22. Veronesi G, Bellomi M, Veronesi U, et al. Role of positron emission tomography scanning in the management of lung nodules detected at baseline computed tomography screening. Ann Thorac Surg 2007;84(3):959–66.
23. Veronesi G, Maisonneuve P, Bellomi M, et al. Estimating overdiagnosis in low-dose computed

tomography screening for lung cancer: a cohort study. Ann Intern Med 2012;157(11):776–84.

24. Maisonneuve P, Bagnardi V, Bellomi M, et al. Lung cancer risk prediction to select smokers for screening CT–a model based on the Italian COSMOS trial. Cancer Prev Res 2011;4(11):1778–89.

25. Maisonneuve P, Casiraghi M, Bertolotti R, et al. P1.04-03 Independent Validation of the Maisonneuve Lung Cancer Risk Model to Optimize Screening Interval in High-risk Individuals. J Thorac Oncol 2022;17(9):S102.

26. Rampinelli C, De Marco P, Origgi D, et al. Exposure to low dose computed tomography for lung cancer screening and risk of cancer: secondary analysis of trial data and risk-benefit analysis. BMJ 2017;356.

27. Duffy SW, Field JK. Mortality Reduction with Low-Dose CT Screening for Lung Cancer. N Engl J Med 2020;382(6):572–3.

28. Kauczor HU, Baird AM, Blum TG, et al. ESR/ERS statement paper on lung cancer screening. Eur Radiol 2020;30(6):3277–94.

29. Crosbie PA, Balata H, Evison M, et al. Implementing lung cancer screening: baseline results from a community-based "Lung Health Check" pilot in deprived areas of Manchester. Thorax 2019;74(4):405–9.

30. Hinde S, Crilly T, Balata H, et al. The cost-effectiveness of the Manchester "lung health checks". a community-based lung cancer low-dose CT screening pilot. Lung Cancer 2018;126:119–24.

31. Black WC, Gareen IF, Soneji SS, et al. Cost-effectiveness of CT screening in the National Lung Screening Trial. N Engl J Med 2014;371(19):1793–802.

32. Postmus PE, Kerr KM, Oudkerk M, et al. Early and locally advanced non-small-cell lung cancer (NSCLC): ESMO Clinical Practice Guidelines for diagnosis, treatment and follow-up. Ann Oncol 2017;28(suppl_4):iv1–21.

33. Pedersen JH, Rzyman W, Veronesi G, et al. Recommendations from the European Society of Thoracic Surgeons (ESTS) regarding computed tomography screening for lung cancer in Europe. Eur J Cardio Thorac Surg 2017;51(3):411–20.

34. Veronesi G, Baldwin DR, Henschke CI, et al. Recommendations for Implementing Lung Cancer Screening with Low-Dose Computed Tomography in Europe. Cancers 2020;12:1672.

35. SAPEA. Cancer screening. Available at: https://sapea.info/topic/cancer-screening/. Accessed March 29, 2023.

36. Pastorino U, Boeri M, Sestini S, et al. Baseline computed tomography screening and blood microRNA predict lung cancer risk and define adequate intervals in the BioMILD trial. Ann Oncol 2022;33(4):395–405.

37. Montani F, Marzi MJ, Dezi F, et al. miR-Test: a blood test for lung cancer early detection. J Natl Cancer Inst 2015;107(6):djv063.

38. Tammemägi MC, Katki HA, Hocking WG, et al. Selection criteria for lung-cancer screening. N Engl J Med 2013;368(8):728–36.

39. Zhao Y, De Bock GH, Vliegenthart R, et al. Performance of computer-aided detection of pulmonary nodules in low-dose CT: comparison with double reading by nodule volume. Eur Radiol 2012;22(10):2076–84.

40. Zhang Y, Jiang B, Zhang L, et al. Lung Nodule Detectability of Artificial Intelligence-assisted CT Image Reading in Lung Cancer Screening. Curr Med Imaging 2022;18(3):327–34.

41. Revel MP, Abdoul H, Chassagnon G, et al. Lung CAncer SCreening in French women using low-dose CT and Artificial intelligence for DEtection: the CASCADE study protocol. BMJ Open 2022;12(12).

Asian Perspective on Lung Cancer Screening

Takahiro Mimae, MD, PhD, Morihito Okada, MD, PhD*

KEYWORDS

- Low-dose computed tomography • Sputum cytology • Chest radiography • Wedge resection
- Segmentectomy

KEY POINTS

- Lung cancer screening (LCS)—not covered by insurance—using low-dose chest computed tomography (CT) for heavy smokers with 30 or more pack-years aged 50 years or older is recommended in Japan because evidence suggests its correlation with lung cancer mortality reduction.
- LCS using low-dose chest CT for nonsmokers/light smokers is not recommended as a countermeasure-type screening because there is insufficient evidence to demonstrate a lung cancer mortality-reducing effect.
- LCS using chest radiography for the non-high-risk group, including nonsmokers/light smokers, and combined chest radiography and sputum cytology for the high-risk group, heavy smokers with 30 or more pack-years aged 50 years or older, is recommended because evidence supports its association with lung cancer mortality reduction in Japan.

INTRODUCTION

Lung cancer is the leading cause of cancer-related mortality in Japan and worldwide.[1,2] In 2021, an estimated 127,400 new cases (85,300 in men and 42,100 in women) of lung and bronchial cancer will be diagnosed, and 74,900 deaths (52,600 in men and 22,300 in women) are estimated to occur in Japan due to the disease, accounting for approximately 20% of all cancer-related deaths.[2] The 5-year relative survival rates for lung cancer are 83.5% for localized disease, 31.1% for regional disease, and 6.4% for distant disease.[3,4] Early detection of lung cancer is an important strategy for decreasing mortality.

The risk factors for the development of lung cancer are well known, especially smoking tobacco.[5,6] Although there is no doubt that smoking cessation is important for the prevention of the development of lung cancers, mere control of smoking is not enough in Japan or Asian countries where many nonsmokers have lung cancer, emphasizing the importance of early detection of lung cancer. Lung cancers in nonsmokers frequently include ground-glass opacity (GGO) on high-resolution computed tomography (HRCT) and are known to show low-grade malignancy. However, even among lung cancers with low-grade malignancy, large tumors show more aggressive behavior than small tumors.[7] In addition, the early identification of small tumors can increase the likelihood of limited resection approaches, such as wedge resection and segmentectomy, and thus increase the provision of timely treatment with a favorable prognosis, not only in younger patients but also in older patients.[8–11]

Advances in diagnostic imaging have made it possible to detect lung cancer at an early stage in medical practice. Conversely, screening of asymptomatic healthy populations is recommended only when the evidence shows the benefits of regular intervention, the reduction of the relevant cancer mortality rate in the examined population outweighs the disadvantages, such as radiation exposure, overdiagnosis, and incidental complications of the detailed examinations. In other words, lung cancer screening (LCS) should (1) improve outcomes; (2) be scientifically

Department of Surgical Oncology, Hiroshima University, 1-2-3 Kasumi, Minami-ku, Hiroshima 734-8551, Japan
* Corresponding author.
E-mail address: morihito@hiroshima-u.ac.jp

Thorac Surg Clin 33 (2023) 385–400
https://doi.org/10.1016/j.thorsurg.2023.03.004
1547-4127/23/© 2023 Elsevier Inc. All rights reserved.

validated; and (3) be a low-risk, reproducible, accessible, and cost-effective strategy.

The National Comprehensive Cancer Network (NCCN) Clinical Practice Guidelines in Oncology (NCCN Guidelines) for LCS were developed in 2011 and are updated every year.[12,13] This article examined the perspective of LCS in Japan, with a focus on the "Lung Cancer Screening Guideline" or "Guidelines for Diagnosis and Treatment of the Lung Cancer/Malignant Pleural Mesothelioma/Thymic Tumors 2022".[14,15]

DECREASE IN LUNG CANCER MORTALITY
Low-Dose Computed Tomography

When computed tomography (CT) examinations are performed for LCS of asymptomatic healthy subjects, the exposure should be reduced as much as possible. Low-dose CT refers to CT with a reduced radiation dose compared with the dose used in CT for general medical examinations. In the past, deterioration of image quality was a problem but many recent studies have resolved the trade-off between radiation dose and image quality, such that even low-dose CT can fully achieve the purpose of LCS. The specific definition of "low dose" in LCS is "imaging conditions that result in a CTDIvol of 2.5 mGy or less in a subject of standard body shape," and low-dose CT imaging should be performed in accordance with this standard.

Previously, low-dose CT was considered to provide insufficient evidence of a mortality-reducing effect, so the rationale for recommending it was unclear. Since then, a series of randomized controlled trials of low-dose CT screening have been conducted in the United States and Europe.[12,16–27] All these studies were included heavy smokers. Of these, the National Lung Screening Trial (NLST) in the United States compared low-dose CT with chest radiography, whereas other randomized controlled trials in Europe compared low-dose CT with no screening or usual care, showing a difference in the control group setting. None of the other randomized controlled trials conducted in Europe showed a significant reduction in lung cancer mortality with low-dose CT screening, except for the Dutch–Belgian lung-cancer screening trial (Nederlands–Leuvens Longkanker Screenings Onderzoek [NELSON])[18] and Multicentric Italian Lung Detection (MILD),[22–24] which showed a significant difference in long-term observations. MILD had an anomalous design, in which a control group was added later and randomization was broken, and it is debatable whether it can be considered to be on par with other randomized controlled trials.

To our knowledge, there are currently no reports of randomized controlled trials to help make decisions for nonsmokers and light smokers. Currently, a randomized controlled trial for these subjects is being conducted in Japan as part of the Japan Agency for Medical Research and Development (AMED) study. This AMED study is a prospective, randomized, controlled phase III study with a total of 27,000 male/female, aged 50 to 70 years, never/light smokers (pack-years ≤30) that aims to compare the lung cancer mortality in the CT group and chest radiography group to verify whether the use of "low-dose CT" as LCS reduces lung cancer death. The CT group was offered low-dose chest CT screening in years 1 and 6, and the chest radiography group was offered chest radiography screening in year 1, with the recommendation that they undergo regular screening in the remaining years and be observed for 10 years. The results of this study are waiting. For heavy smokers, 2 large randomized controlled trials[12,16,22–25] in different regions showed a significant reduction in lung cancer mortality in the low-dose CT screening group as compared with the control group. However, there are many differences among studies in the scale of randomization and sample size, the setting of the CT screening control group; age, sex, and smoking history of the subjects to be screened; and the interval between low-dose CT examinations. Meta-analyses[28,29] including these trials have shown a reduction in lung cancer mortality, and examination of heterogeneity in 2 independent meta-analyses did not detect a problematic level of heterogeneity. The US Preventive Services Task Force's systematic review,[30] which does not include a meta-analysis but rather a summary of previous studies, posits that low-dose CT screening is effective in reducing lung cancer mortality. Although no randomized controlled trials have been conducted in Japan for heavy smokers, the results of randomized controlled trials and meta-analyses conducted in several countries suggest that low-dose CT screening for heavy smokers is likely to be effective in Japan (Table 1).[15] However, insufficient evidence supports lung cancer mortality reduction with the use of LCS in nonsmokers and light smokers. Thus far, the target population for LCS in Japan has been defined as men and women aged 50 years or older with pack-years of 30 or higher based on the results of the NLST/NELSON trials, consistent with the high-risk population defined in the current Japanese LCS system.

Other Screening Modalities

In Japan, chest radiography for non-high-risk patients and combined chest radiography and

Table 1
Criteria and guidance classifications of low-dose computed tomography scan based on Lung Cancer Screening Guideline in Japan

Temporary Classification by Double Interpretation	Final Classification After Comparative Interpretation	Low-Dose CT Findings	Temporary Guidance by Double Interpretation	Final Guidance after Comparative Interpretation
a	A	"Impossible to interpret" Due to inappropriate imaging condition, inappropriate position, and artifact	Reimaging	
b	B	"No abnormality" Including normal variant	Regular low-dose CT screening	
c	C	"Abnormality without the necessity of detailed examination" <6-mm nodule, as average of maximum and minimum diameter. No need for detailed examination or treatment due to old change, calcification, fibrosis, bronchiectatic dilatations, emphysematous changes, postoperative changes, malformations that do not require treatment, and so forth		
d	D	"Abnormal findings and possible conditions other than lung cancer requiring treatment" Suspicion of a disease other than lung cancer that would be detrimental to the patient and those around him/her if a detailed examination and treatment are not performed urgently. Classify "C" for suspicion of a disease not requiring a detailed examination and urgent treatment. Classify "E" if there is suspicion of lung cancer, even slightly. "Screening positive" as lung cancer screening is only "E"	Comparative interpretation	Detailed examination for applicable diseases other than lung cancer
d1	D1	"Active pulmonary tuberculosis" Suspicion of tuberculosis requiring treatment		Detailed examination for lung cancer
d2	D2	"Active nontuberculous lung disease" Suspicion of conditions such as pneumonia and pneumothorax requiring treatment		
d3	D3	"Cardiovascular disease" Suspicion of cardiovascular anomaly such as aortic aneurysm requiring treatment		

(continued on next page)

Table 1
(continued)

Temporary Classification by Double Interpretation	Final Classification After Comparative Interpretation	Low-Dose CT Findings	Temporary Guidance by Double Interpretation	Final Guidance after Comparative Interpretation
d4	D4	"Others" Suspicion of conditions including mediastinal tumors, chest wall tumor, pleural tumor, and so forth requiring treatment		
e	E	"Suspicion of lung cancer" ≥6-mm nodule, as average of maximum and minimum diameter, secondary changes due to lung cancer such as pleural effusion, atelectasis, and so forth		
e1	E1	"Suspicion of lung cancer cannot be ruled out"		
e2	E2	"Strong suspicion of lung cancer"		

1. In final guidance after comparative interpretation, "E1" means suspicion of lung cancer, even if slight, and "E2" means strong suspicion of lung cancer. However, "D" means suspicion of a disease other than lung cancer.
2. Person requiring detailed examination on low-dose CT as lung cancer screening is classified as "E1" or "E2" on final guidance after comparative interpretation.
3. "D" on final guidance after comparative interpretation does not mean person requiring detailed examination on lung cancer screening.
4. The number of persons requiring detailed examination on low-dose CT as lung cancer screening means the total number of "E1" and "E2."
5. The number of patients diagnosed with lung cancer, that is, lung cancer detected by screening, on lung cancer screening means the number of patients definitely diagnosed with lung cancer among persons requiring detailed examination based on classification of "E1" or "E2."
6. Lung cancer detected in persons classified as "D" does not correspond lung cancer detected by screening.
7. Detailed examination for lung cancer in a person classified as "E" on final guidance after comparative interpretation conforms to "Concept of Criteria and Follow-up for Lung Nodules on Lung Cancer Screening with low-dose CT" edited by Lung Cancer Diagnostic Criteria Subcommittee, The Japanese Society of CT screening.
Modified from Lung Cancer Screening Guideline of General Rule for Clinical and Pathological Record of Lung Cancer. 8th ed, revised version.

sputum cytology for high-risk patients are recommended because there is reasonable evidence of a lung cancer mortality-reducing effect with these strategies. However, these practices should be carried out only if standard interpretation methods, including double interpretation and comparative interpretation, are used (**Fig. 1, Tables 2** and **3**).[15] Double interpretation is a method of maintaining accuracy by having 2 physicians diagnose a single chest radiograph separately to prevent overinterpretation or underinterpretation. These are referred to as the primary and secondary interpretations. When an abnormality is found on a chest radiographic scan, the previous chest scan is examined in detail alongside the scan on which the abnormality was found. This comparison of the same patient's previous and present scans is called comparative interpretation.

Chest radiographs for the non-high-risk group and combined chest radiography and sputum cytology for the high-risk group have been shown to significantly reduce lung cancer mortality in 4 case-control studies in Japan.[31–34] No significant mortality reduction in lung cancer was observed in 2 previous randomized controlled studies conducted in the United States and Europe.[35–37] Case-control studies are observational and cannot completely control for bias, including self-selection bias. However, the randomized controlled trials in Europe and the United States are very old, the standard of medical care referred to in those trials is different from the standards adopted at present, there may be racial differences, and the control of compliance and contamination may have been inadequate. Considering these factors, 5 case-control studies (**Table 4**)[31–34,38] from Japan showed generally the same trend, 4 of which were significant—they retained the trend of lung cancer mortality reduction despite various attempts to eliminate the effects of bias; therefore, it is appropriate to focus on the reports from Japan as evidence to be used for the LCS guidelines in modern Japan. The districts in which the lung cancer mortality reduction effect was observed might have been influenced by the use of standard methods, including double interpretation and comparative interpretation, and in the districts where such methods were not used, the effect was not significant. In addition, sufficient explanation of disadvantages such as radiation exposure, false-negatives, false-positives, overdiagnosis, and the risks of close examination should be provided in advance.

A case-control study on the effect of chest radiography alone on lung cancer mortality reduction did not show a significant result.[39–41] However, sputum cytology is the only screening method for early lung cancer in the hilar region that is noninvasive and easy to perform. The detection sensitivity

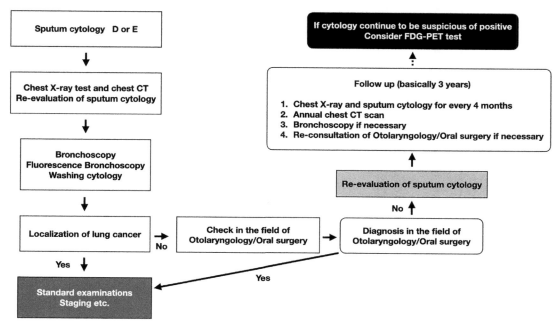

Fig. 1. Detailed examination procedures for a person with sputum cytology classification D or E as well as abnormal findings and possible conditions other than lung cancer or suspected to be lung cancer, requiring treatment. FDG-PET, [(18)F] Fluorodeoxyglucose-positron emission tomography. (*From* Lung Cancer Screening Guideline of General Rule for Clinical and Pathological Record of Lung Cancer. 8th ed, revised version.)

Table 2
Criteria and guidance classifications of chest radiography based on Lung Cancer Screening Guideline in Japan

Temporary Classification by Double Interpretation	Final Classification After Comparative Interpretation	Chest Radiography Findings	Temporary Guidance by Double Interpretation	Final Guidance After Comparative Interpretation
a	A	"Impossible to interpret" Due to inappropriate imaging condition, inappropriate position, film scratches, and artifact	Reimaging	
b	B	"No abnormality" Including normal variant such as parapericardial adipose tissue, tent-like and vault-shaped deformity of the diaphragm, associated shadows due to subpleural adipose tissue, shadow of the right cardiac border	Regular screening	
c	C	"Abnormality without the necessity of detailed examination" No necessity of detailed examination or treatment due to old age, calcification, fibrosis, bronchiectatic dilatations, emphysematous changes, postoperative changes, malformations that do not require treatment, and so forth		

			Comparative interpretation	
d	D	"Abnormal findings and possible conditions other than lung cancer requiring treatment" Suspicious of a disease other than lung cancer that would be of treat detriment to the patient and those around him/her if a detailed examination and treatment are not performed urgently. Classify "C" for suspicion of a disease not requiring a detailed examination and urgent treatment. Classify "E" if there is even slight suspicion of lung cancer. "Screening positive" as lung cancer screening is only "E."		Detailed examination for applicable diseases other than lung cancer
d1	D1	"Active pulmonary tuberculosis" Suspicion of tuberculosis requiring treatment		Detailed examination for lung cancer
d2	D2	"Active nontuberculous lung disease" Suspicion of conditions such as pneumonia and pneumothorax requiring treatment		
d3	D3	"Cardiovascular disease" Suspicion of cardiovascular anomaly such as aortic aneurysm requiring treatment		

(continued on next page)

Table 2
(continued)

Temporary Classification by Double Interpretation	Final Classification After Comparative Interpretation	Chest Radiography Findings	Temporary Guidance by Double Interpretation	Final Guidance After Comparative Interpretation
d4	D4	"Others" Suspicion of conditions including mediastinal tumors, chest wall tumor, pleural tumor, and so forth requiring treatment		
e	E	"Suspicion of lung cancer" New shadow on solitary shadow/old change, abnormality such as mass shadow and shift in hilar structures including vascular/bronchus, secondary changes such as pneumonia and atelectasis due to stenosis/obstruction of bronchus, other findings suspicious of lung cancer. Accordingly, "E" includes a part of pneumonia and pleuritis. Classify "E" if suspicious of metastatic lung tumor. (However, metastatic lung tumor is not included as lung cancer detected by screening.) In case of "E2," strongly encourage the patient to undergo a detailed examination as soon as possible		
e1	E1	"Suspicion of lung cancer cannot be ruled out"		
e2	E2	"Strong suspicion of lung cancer"		

1. In final guidance after comparative interpretation, "E1" means suspicion of lung cancer, even if slight, and "E2" means strong suspicion of lung cancer. However, "D" means suspicion of a disease other than lung cancer.

2. Person requiring detailed examination on chest radiography for lung cancer screening is classified as "E1" or "E2" on final guidance after comparative interpretation.

3. "D" on final guidance after comparative interpretation does not mean person requiring detailed examination on lung cancer screening.

4. The number of persons requiring detailed examination on chest radiography for lung cancer screening means the total number of "E1" and "E2."

5. The number of patients diagnosed with lung cancer, that is, lung cancer detected by screening, on lung cancer screening means the number of patients definitely diagnosed with lung cancer among persons requiring detailed examination based on classification of "E1" or "E2."

6. Lung cancer detected in persons classified as "D" does not correspond lung cancer detected by screening.

Modified from Lung Cancer Screening Guideline of General Rule for Clinical and Pathologic Record of Lung Cancer. 8th ed, revised version.

Table 3
Criteria and guidance classifications of sputum cytology based on Lung Cancer Screening Guideline in Japan

Classification	Cytology Findings	Guidance
A	No histiocytes in sputum	Inappropriate material, reexamination
B	Only normal epithelial cells Basal cells proliferation Mild atypical squamous cells Ciliated columnar epithelial cells	No abnormalities at present Next routine examination
C	Moderate atypical squamous cells Columnar epithelial cells with enlargement/deep dyeing of nuclei	Resmear or reexamination within 6 mo
D	Highly/border atypical squamous cells or suspicious of malignant cells	Immediate detailed examination
E	Malignant cells	

1. A comprehensive judgment is made based on all specimens of one sputum sample but reexamination should be considered in cases with a small number of atypical cells.
2. Determined by the highest degree of cellular atypia on the whole specimen.
3. The atypicality of squamous cells is determined by referring to the criteria for atypical squamous cells and cytology chart.
4. If reexamination is difficult, next routine examination is recommended.
5. Whenever no cancer is detected because of a detailed examination due to d/E classification, the patient is followed closely.
Modified from Lung Cancer Screening Guideline of General Rule for Clinical and Pathologic Record of Lung Cancer. 8th ed, revised version.

of sputum cytology in lung cancer cases is only approximately 40%[42]; however, radiograph-negative lung cancers detected by sputum cytology are reportedly associated with a high rate of long-term survival.[43] In randomized controlled trials that examined the effectiveness of a screening method in which sputum cytology was added to chest radiography, namely the Johns Hopkins Study[44] and Memorial Sloan-Kettering Study,[36] the rate of early stage cancer, resection rate, and 5-year survival rate increased in the group in which sputum cytology was added. In a mixed analysis of long-term follow-up in both studies, a trend toward a 12% reduction in mortality was observed but the difference between the groups was not statistically significant.[45] The results of a joint survey by the Japan Lung Cancer Society, Japanese Society of Clinical Cytology, and Japan Society for Respiratory Endoscopy also showed that sputum cytology was effective in detecting hilar lung cancer.[46] Although the detection rate of sputum cytology is low and there is little evidence of the effectiveness of this technique, it is a simple and noninvasive test and is considered important in the detection of hilar lung cancer in high-risk groups, such as those aged 50 years or older with 30 or more pack-years.

The detection sensitivity of PET/CT for lung cancer is approximately 83% to 96%, with a specificity of 78% to 91%[47,48] but the sensitivity is reduced for stage I disease.[49,50] PET/CT produce false-negative results for small lesions less than 10 mm in diameter and histologically low-grade lesions. PET/CT also produces false-positives in cases of nonneoplastic disease.[49] Conversely, a meta-analysis showed that PET/CT tended to be superior to chest radiography and CT for the positive diagnosis of pulmonary nodules, although the difference was not significant.[51,52] Therefore, PET/CT is not intended for the detection of lung cancer but as an adjunct to the qualitative and staging diagnosis of lung nodules. PET/CT is not recommended as LCS.

Serum tumor markers alone do not improve lung cancer detection rates because they can lead to false-negative or false-positive findings.[53] The sensitivity of serum cytokeratin 19 fragment antigen 21-1 (CYFRA21-1) in detecting non-small cell carcinoma ranges from 41% to 65%, and the sensitivities of serum carcinoembryonic antigen, sialyl Lex-i antigen, carbohydrate Antigen 19-9 (CA19-9), carbohydrate Antigen 125 (CA125), squamous cell carcinoma antigen, and tissue polypeptide antigen are lower than that of CYFRA21-1 but these values vary depending on the histologic type and stage.[54–56] The combination of multiple tumor markers has also been reported to improve detection sensitivity.[57,58] However, most studies on

Table 4
Comparison of 5 case-control studies

Study	Okayama Study	Kanagawa Study	Miyagi Study	Niigata Study	JLCSRG
Study design	Matched CC	Matched CC	Matched CC	Matched CC	Matched CC
Screening methods	Annual (CXp/SpC)	Annual (CXp/SpC)	Annual (CXp/SpC)	Annual (CXp/SpC)	Annual (CXp/SpC)
Source population	Those who were invited to the screening	National health insurance holders	Examinees with previous negative result	National health insurance holders	Depend on the areas (Those who were invited to the screening/National health insurance holders)
Case	Decedent from lung cancer at the age of 40–79 y	Decedent from lung cancer at the age of 40–74 y	Decedent from lung cancer at the age of 40–79 y	Decedent from lung cancer at the age of 40–79 y	Decedent from lung cancer at the age of 40–79 y
Case:control	1:10	1:3	1:6	1:5	1:2–5
Matching condition	Sex, year of birth, and municipality	Sex, year of birth, and municipality	Sex, year of birth, municipality, and smoking habit	Sex, year of birth, municipality, and smoking habit	Sex, age, smoking status and type of health insurance
Source of information about smoking	Interview, medical records, and previous screening records	Medical records and questionnaire	Declaration at previous screening in 1989	Interview and medical records	Interview, screening records, and medical records
Analytical method	LRA	LRA	LRA	LRA	LRA
Adjustment	Smoking index	Smoking index	Smoking index	Smoking index	Smoking index
Number of the cases	412	193	328	174	273
Number of the controls	3490	579	1886	801	1269
Smoking adjusted odds ratio (95%CI)	0.59 (0.46–0.74)	0.54 (0.34–0.85)	0.54 (0.41–0.73)	0.40 (0.27–0.59)	0.72 (0.50–1.03)

Abbreviations: CXp/SpC, chest radiography for all examinees and additional sputum cytology for high-risk examinees; JLCSRG, Japanese Lung-Cancer-Screening Research Group; LRA, logistic regression analysis; Matched CC, matched case-control study; OR, ORs of death from lung cancer among those screened vs unscreened within 12 months before the reference date.

Refer to Sagawa M, et. al. Lung Cancer. 2003;41:29-36.[64]

tumor markers are retrospective in nature in cases of suspected lung cancer by imaging diagnosis or confirmed lung cancer by pathologic diagnosis, and they do not aim to detect tumor markers alone. Therefore, serum tumor markers may be used as an adjunct to the qualitative diagnosis of lung cancer, for monitoring treatment efficacy, and for the diagnosis of recurrence rather than for detecting lung cancer.

Overdiagnosis on Lung Cancer Screening

LCS is performed to detect lung cancer in its early stages and promote effective treatment, with the aim of preventing mortality from lung cancer. Lung cancer progresses over time, eventually resulting in death. However, some lung cancers are not fatal, such as GGO-dominant tumors on HRCT, even if they are not detected on LCS. In other words, in some cases, death from other causes occurs before death from lung cancer. Overdiagnosis on LCS refers to the detection of early stage lung cancer that does not directly lead to death. Overdiagnosis is more likely to occur when the target disease is very slow-growing or in the very early stage or when the person being screened is elderly or has other serious diseases. When a full examination or treatment, including surgery, is performed for lung cancer that does not lead to death, it may contribute to a reduction in the lung cancer mortality rate but it places patients at risk of unnecessary interventions and treatment complications and imposes unnecessary psychological and financial burdens on the patients. Therefore, overdiagnosis is considered one of the disadvantages of LCS.

It is difficult to estimate the overdiagnosis rate or to compare the rates across modalities; however, is important to note that the overdiagnosis rate with LCS is approximately 10% to 40%, even among Western heavy smokers. For Asians including Japanese and nonsmokers, the overdiagnosis rate may be much higher, depending on how the CT screening is performed. Cancer screening is performed to detect cancer while it is asymptomatic to ensure early treatment and prevent mortality. However, the higher the rate of overdiagnosis, the greater the rate of disadvantage to the examinee owing to a series of tests and treatments for cancer that does not lead to death and the associated adverse events and financial and psychological burdens. To reduce the disadvantages of overdiagnosis, it is necessary to consider the criteria for detailed examination and restrictions pertaining to the target group of examinees, target age, and pack-years.

Therefore, examinations that deviate from these criteria should not be conducted. If the diagnosis of lung cancer is histologically confirmed, it is difficult to not consider surgical treatment. However, if early stage lung cancer or suspicious lung cancer nodules are detected on LCS, such as tumors with GGO component on HRCT, follow-up should be aggressively considered without necessarily performing surgery.[59] A prospective study is currently underway as Japan Clinical Oncology Group 1906 to verify this point. This multi-institutional, single-arm confirmatory trial was launched in June 2020 to evaluate the efficacy and safety of watchful waiting for patients with radiologically noninvasive lung cancer, defined as nodules 2 cm or less with a consolidation/tumor ratio of 0.25 or less on HRCT and to provide high-quality information about the optimal timing of surgical intervention for such indolent cancers. A total of 720 patients will be enrolled from 49 institutions during a 5-year period with a primary endpoint of 10-year overall survival.[60]

False-Positive Findings on Lung Cancer Screening

False-positives are defined as positive screening results that are followed before the next screening visit in the case of multiple visits by a thorough examination, for example, CT scan or biopsy, that do not result in a diagnosis of lung cancer. False-positive results should be interpreted with caution because the results vary widely depending on the study design and the definition of "positive nodule," including the nodule size threshold (eg, whether the diameter is 4, 5, or 6 mm), the use of volume doubling time, and features of the nodule, such as pure solid, part-solid/mixed GGO, or pure GGO.

Two systematic reviews of low-dose CT screening studies reported on false-positives.[30,61] Ali and colleagues examined the frequency of false-positives separately for single and multiple examinations.[61] In single examinations, 7,619 of 30,536 participants yielded false-positives findings (median, 25.53%; range, 7.90%–26.23%). For multiple screenings, 8,469 of 43,943 participants had at least one false-positive finding (median, 23.28%; range, 0.64%–69.0%). The report by Jonas and colleagues is a large systematic review of 27 studies.[30] The false-positive rates ranged 7.9% to 49.3% for first-time examinations and 0.6% to 28.6% for second and subsequent examinations. As mentioned earlier, the different ranges of false-positive rates were observed because of the different definitions of a positive nodule used in different studies.

A systematic review[61] summarizing 2 randomized controlled trials[12,62] and one cohort study[63] of false-positives on chest radiography reported that of the 33,199 participants screened multiple times, 2,098 had at least one false-positive result (median, 6.50%, range 3.40%–13.67%). In the NLST,[12] the largest randomized controlled trial, the false-positive rates were 8.6%, 5.9%, and 4.7% at the first year, at 1 year, and at 2 years, respectively.

Some nodules that test positive are subjected to invasive procedures, such as needle biopsy or thoracoscopic biopsy, and serious complications may occur, although infrequently. False-positive cases that cannot be diagnosed require long-term follow-up with imaging studies. However, radiation exposure is also a problem. False-positive results are one of the important "disadvantage" of screening. In a population with a preponderance of true-negatives, the false-positive rate is almost equal to the rate of those who require further examination. It is necessary to optimize the screening process to minimize the false-positive rate as much as possible without increasing the number of false-negative cases, considering the use of artificial intelligence and other modalities; further research on the risk assessment of negative results is needed.

SUMMARY

LCS using low-dose chest CT for heavy smokers with 30 or more pack-years aged 50 years or older is recommended because there is evidence of LCS reducing the lung cancer mortality in this patient group. However, LCS should be performed only when it is conducted using a reliable accuracy control system. It is not recommended under an inadequate accuracy control system, such as a low screening uptake rate or inadequate tracking of those who need to be examined further.

LCS using chest radiography for the non-high-risk group and combined chest radiography and sputum cytology for the high-risk group, that is, heavy smokers with 30 or more pack-years aged 50 years or older, is recommended because there is evidence of LCS reducing lung cancer mortality in this patient group in the context of Japan. However, LCS should be carried out only if standard interpretation methods, including double interpretation and comparative interpretation, are used. Future studies should examine the need for thorough accuracy control and nationwide equalization as well as sensitivity and specificity of LCS and the extent of its contribution to nationwide reduction in lung cancer mortality.

CLINICS CARE POINTS

- Low-dose CT should be selected for LCS but not non-low-dose CT because of the risk of radiation exposure.
- When detecting the lesions suspicious of lung cancer on LCS, the double interpretation or the comparative interpretation is important to conclude the necessity of the detailed examination.
- Ground glass opacity dominant nodule, often detected on LCS in Asian countries, should be determined if the treatment of the lesion is immediately necessary under consideration of overdiagnosis.

DISCLOSURE

This study was supported by grants from the Japan Society for the Promotion of Science (JSPS), Japan KAKENHI, Japan (20K09177).

CONFLICT OF INTERESTS

The authors have nothing to disclose.

REFERENCES

1. Torre LA, Siegel RL, Ward EM, et al. Global cancer incidence and mortality rates and trends–an update. Cancer Epidemiol Biomarkers Prev 2016;25:16–27.
2. Cancer Statistics. Cancer Information Service, National Cancer Center, Japan (Vital Statistics of Japan, Ministry of Health, Labour and Welfare). Available at: https://ganjoho.jp/public/qa_links/report/statistics/2022_jp.html. Accessed 10 January, 2023.
3. Matsuda T, Ajiki W, Marugame T, et al. Population-based survival of cancer patients diagnosed between 1993 and 1999 in Japan: a chronological and international comparative study. Jpn J Clin Oncol 2011;41:40–51.
4. Monitoring of Cancer Incidence in Japan - Survival 2009-2011 Report (Center for Cancer Control and Information Services, National Cancer Center, 2020). Available at: https://ganjoho.jp/reg_stat/statistics/data/dl/index.html. Accessed 10 January, 2023.
5. Jemal A, Thun MJ, Ries LA, et al. Annual report to the nation on the status of cancer, 1975-2005, featuring trends in lung cancer, tobacco use, and tobacco control. J Natl Cancer Inst 2008;100:1672–94.
6. Jemal A, Ward EM, Johnson CJ, et al. Annual Report to the Nation on the Status of Cancer, 1975-2014,

Featuring Survival. J Natl Cancer Inst 2017;109(9): djx030.

7. Mimae T, Tsutani Y, Miyata Y, et al. Solid tumor size of 2 cm divides outcomes of patients with mixed ground glass opacity lung tumors. Ann Thorac Surg 2020;109:1530–6.

8. Mimae T, Miyata Y, Tsutani Y, et al. Wedge resection as an alternative treatment for octogenarian and older patients with early-stage non-small-cell lung cancer. Jpn J Clin Oncol 2020;50:1051–7.

9. Mimae T, Okada M. Are segmentectomy and lobectomy comparable in terms of curative intent for early stage non-small cell lung cancer? Gen Thorac Cardiovasc Surg 2020;68:703–6.

10. Mimae T, Saji H, Nakamura H, et al. Survival of octogenarians with early-stage non-small cell lung cancer is comparable between wedge resection and lobectomy/segmentectomy: JACS1303. Ann Surg Oncol 2021;28:7219–27.

11. Saji H, Okada M, Tsuboi M, et al. Segmentectomy versus lobectomy in small-sized peripheral non-small-cell lung cancer (JCOG0802/WJOG4607L): a multicentre, open-label, phase 3, randomised, controlled, non-inferiority trial. Lancet 2022;399: 1607–17.

12. Aberle DR, Adams AM, Berg CD, et al. Reduced lung-cancer mortality with low-dose computed tomographic screening. N Engl J Med 2011;365: 395–409.

13. Wood DE, Kazerooni EA, Aberle D, et al. NCCN Guidelines® Insights: Lung Cancer Screening, Version 1.2022. J Natl Compr Canc Netw 2022;20: 754–64.

14. The Japan Lung Cancer Society. Guidelines for Diagnosis and Treatment of the Lung Cancer/Malignant Pleural Mesothelioma/Thymic Tumors 2022. Available at: https://www.haigan.gr.jp/guideline/2022/. Accessed 8 January, 2023.

15. The Japan Lung Cancer Society. General Rule for clinical and pathological Record of lung cancer. 8th Edition. Tokyo: KANEHARA; 2021. p. 187–212.

16. National Lung Screening Trial Research Team. Lung Cancer Incidence and Mortality with Extended Follow-up in the National Lung Screening Trial. J Thorac Oncol 2019;14:1732–42.

17. Becker N, Motsch E, Trotter A, et al. Lung cancer mortality reduction by LDCT screening-Results from the randomized German LUSI trial. Int J Cancer 2020;146:1503–13.

18. de Koning HJ, van der Aalst CM, de Jong PA, et al. Reduced lung-cancer mortality with volume CT screening in a randomized trial. N Engl J Med 2020;382:503–13.

19. Field JK, Vulkan D, Davies MPA, et al. Lung cancer mortality reduction by LDCT screening: UKLS randomised trial results and international meta-analysis. Lancet Reg Health Eur 2021;10:100179.

20. Infante M, Cavuto S, Lutman FR, et al. Long-term follow-up results of the DANTE Trial, a randomized study of lung cancer screening with spiral computed tomography. Am J Respir Crit Care Med 2015;191: 1166–75.

21. Paci E, Puliti D, Lopes Pegna A, et al. Mortality, survival and incidence rates in the ITALUNG randomised lung cancer screening trial. Thorax 2017;72: 825–31.

22. Pastorino U, Rossi M, Rosato V, et al. Annual or biennial CT screening versus observation in heavy smokers: 5-year results of the MILD trial. Eur J Cancer Prev 2012;21:308–15.

23. Pastorino U, Silva M, Sestini S, et al. Prolonged lung cancer screening reduced 10-year mortality in the MILD trial: new confirmation of lung cancer screening efficacy. Ann Oncol 2019;30:1162–9.

24. Pastorino U, Sverzellati N, Sestini S, et al. Ten-year results of the Multicentric Italian Lung Detection trial demonstrate the safety and efficacy of biennial lung cancer screening. Eur J Cancer 2019;118:142–8.

25. Pinsky PF, Church TR, Izmirlian G, et al. The National Lung Screening Trial: results stratified by demographics, smoking history, and lung cancer histology. Cancer 2013;119:3976–83.

26. Saghir Z, Dirksen A, Ashraf H, et al. CT screening for lung cancer brings forward early disease. The randomised Danish Lung Cancer Screening Trial: status after five annual screening rounds with low-dose CT. Thorax 2012;67:296–301.

27. Wille MM, Dirksen A, Ashraf H, et al. Results of the randomized Danish Lung Cancer Screening Trial with focus on high-risk profiling. Am J Respir Crit Care Med 2016;193:542–51.

28. Huang KL, Wang SY, Lu WC, et al. Effects of low-dose computed tomography on lung cancer screening: a systematic review, meta-analysis, and trial sequential analysis. BMC Pulm Med 2019;19: 126.

29. Sadate A, Occean BV, Beregi JP, et al. Systematic review and meta-analysis on the impact of lung cancer screening by low-dose computed tomography. Eur J Cancer 2020;134:107–14.

30. Jonas DE, Reuland DS, Reddy SM, et al. Screening for lung cancer with low-dose computed tomography: updated evidence report and systematic review for the US Preventive Services Task Force. JAMA 2021;325:971–87.

31. Nishii K, Ueoka H, Kiura K, et al. A case-control study of lung cancer screening in Okayama Prefecture, Japan. Lung Cancer 2001;34:325–32.

32. Okamoto N, Suzuki T, Hasegawa H, et al. Evaluation of a clinic-based screening program for lung cancer with a case-control design in Kanagawa, Japan. Lung Cancer 1999;25:77–85.

33. Sagawa M, Tsubono Y, Saito Y, et al. A case-control study for evaluating the efficacy of mass screening

program for lung cancer in Miyagi Prefecture, Japan. Cancer 2001;92:588–94.

34. Tsukada H, Kurita Y, Yokoyama A, et al. An evaluation of screening for lung cancer in Niigata Prefecture, Japan: a population-based case-control study. Br J Cancer 2001;85:1326–31.

35. Melamed MR, Flehinger BJ. Detection of lung cancer: highlights of the Memorial Sloan-Kettering Study in New York City. Schweiz Med Wochenschr 1987;117:1457–63.

36. Melamed MR, Flehinger BJ, Zaman MB, et al. Screening for early lung cancer. Results of the Memorial Sloan-Kettering study in New York. Chest 1984;86:44–53.

37. Strauss GM, Gleason RE, Sugarbaker DJ. Screening for lung cancer. Another look; a different view. Chest 1997;111:754–68.

38. Sobue T, Suzuki T, Naruke T. A case-control study for evaluating lung-cancer screening in Japan. Japanese Lung-Cancer-Screening Research Group. Int J Cancer 1992;50:230–7.

39. Berndt R, Nischan P, Ebeling K. Screening for lung cancer in the middle-aged. Int J Cancer 1990;45:229–30.

40. Ebeling K, Nischan P. Screening for lung cancer—results from a case-control study. Int J Cancer 1987;40:141–4.

41. Nakayama T, Baba T, Suzuki T, et al. An evaluation of chest X-ray screening for lung cancer in Gunma prefecture, Japan: a population-based case-control study. Eur J Cancer 2002;38:1380–7.

42. Sing A, Freudenberg N, Kortsik C, et al. Comparison of the sensitivity of sputum and brush cytology in the diagnosis of lung carcinomas. Acta Cytol 1997;41:399–408.

43. Bechtel JJ, Petty TL, Saccomanno G. Five year survival and later outcome of patients with X-ray occult lung cancer detected by sputum cytology. Lung Cancer 2000;30:1–7.

44. Frost JK, Ball WC Jr, Levin ML, et al. Early lung cancer detection: results of the initial (prevalence) radiologic and cytologic screening in the Johns Hopkins study. Am Rev Respir Dis 1984;130:549–54.

45. Doria-Rose VP, Marcus PM, Szabo E, et al. Randomized controlled trials of the efficacy of lung cancer screening by sputum cytology revisited: a combined mortality analysis from the Johns Hopkins Lung Project and the Memorial Sloan-Kettering Lung Study. Cancer 2009;115:5007–17.

46. Sato M, Saito Y, Kiyoshi Shibuya K, et al. Early Hilar Type Lung Cancer in Japan: A Survey from January 2006 to December 2007. Japanese J Lung Cancer 2011;51:777–86.

47. Chien CR, Liang JA, Chen JH, et al. [(18)F]Fluorodeoxyglucose-positron emission tomography screening for lung cancer: a systematic review and meta-analysis. Cancer Imag 2013;13:458–65.

48. Gould MK, Maclean CC, Kuschner WG, et al. Accuracy of positron emission tomography for diagnosis of pulmonary nodules and mass lesions: a meta-analysis. JAMA 2001;285:914–24.

49. Grogan EL, Deppen SA, Ballman KV, et al. Accuracy of fluorodeoxyglucose-positron emission tomography within the clinical practice of the American College of Surgeons Oncology Group Z4031 trial to diagnose clinical stage I non-small cell lung cancer. Ann Thorac Surg 2014;97:1142–8.

50. Minamimoto R, Senda M, Jinnouchi S, et al. Detection of lung cancer by FDG-PET cancer screening program: a nationwide Japanese survey. Anticancer Res 2014;34:183–9.

51. Cronin P, Dwamena BA, Kelly AM, et al. Solitary pulmonary nodules and masses: a meta-analysis of the diagnostic utility of alternative imaging tests. Eur Radiol 2008;18:1840–56.

52. Cronin P, Dwamena BA, Kelly AM, et al. Solitary pulmonary nodules: meta-analytic comparison of cross-sectional imaging modalities for diagnosis of malignancy. Radiology 2008;246:772–82.

53. Bates SE. Clinical applications of serum tumor markers. Ann Intern Med 1991;115:623–38.

54. Bombardieri E, Seregni E, Bogni A, et al. Evaluation of cytokeratin 19 serum fragments (CYFRA 21-1) in patients with lung cancer: results of a multicenter trial. Int J Biol Markers 1994;9:89–95.

55. Pujol JL, Grenier J, Parrat E, et al. Cytokeratins as serum markers in lung cancer: a comparison of CYFRA 21-1 and TPS. Am J Respir Crit Care Med 1996;154:725–33.

56. Rastel D, Ramaioli A, Cornillie F, et al. CYFRA 21-1, a sensitive and specific new tumour marker for squamous cell lung cancer. Report of the first European multicentre evaluation. CYFRA 21-1 Multicentre Study Group. Eur J Cancer 1994;30a:601–6.

57. Jia H, Zhang L, Wang B. The value of combination analysis of tumor biomarkers for early differentiating diagnosis of lung cancer and pulmonary tuberculosis. Ann Clin Lab Sci 2019;49:645–9.

58. Korkmaz ET, Koksal D, Aksu F, et al. Triple test with tumor markers CYFRA 21.1, HE4, and ProGRP might contribute to diagnosis and subtyping of lung cancer. Clin Biochem 2018;58:15–9.

59. Mimae T, Miyata Y, Tsutani Y, et al. What are the radiologic findings predictive of indolent lung adenocarcinoma? Jpn J Clin Oncol 2015;45:367–72.

60. Miyoshi T, Aokage K, Wakabayashi M, et al. Prospective evaluation of watchful waiting for early-stage lung cancer with ground-glass opacity: a single-arm confirmatory multicenter study: Japan Clinical Oncology Group study JCOG1906 (EVERGREEN study). Jpn J Clin Oncol 2021;51:1330–3.

61. Usman Ali M, Miller J, Peirson L, et al. Screening for lung cancer: A systematic review and meta-analysis. Prev Med 2016;89:301–14.

62. Croswell JM, Baker SG, Marcus PM, et al. Cumulative incidence of false-positive test results in lung cancer screening: a randomized trial. Ann Intern Med 2010;152(505–12):w176–80.

63. Dominioni L, Rotolo N, Mantovani W, et al. A population-based cohort study of chest x-ray screening in smokers: lung cancer detection findings and follow-up. BMC Cancer 2012;12:18.

64. Sagawa M, Nakayama T, Tsukada H, et al. The efficacy of lung cancer screening conducted in 1990s: four case-control studies in Japan. Lung Cancer 2003;41:29–36.

Artificial Intelligence and Machine Learning in Lung Cancer Screening

Scott J. Adams, MD, PhD[a], Peter Mikhael, BSc[b,c], Jeremy Wohlwend, ME[b,c], Regina Barzilay, PhD[b,c], Lecia V. Sequist, MD, MPH[d,e,*], Florian J. Fintelmann, MD[e,f,*]

KEYWORDS

- Lung cancer screening • Artificial intelligence • Machine learning • Risk prediction
- Lung nodule detection • Opportunistic screening

KEY POINTS

- Recent advances in artificial intelligence and machine learning (AI/ML) hold substantial promise to address some of the current challenges in lung cancer screening and improve health equity.
- AI/ML tools have shown predictive ability to identify individuals who would most benefit from screening, which could further improve the efficiency of lung cancer screening programs.
- Currently available AI/ML tools have shown promise to increase sensitivity and specificity for lung nodule detection and classification, which may reduce false positives and unnecessary follow-up investigations and facilitate earlier lung cancer diagnoses.
- The assessment of sarcopenia, cardiovascular disease, and osteoporosis on low-dose chest computed tomography with AI/ML tools creates opportunities to improve population health through opportunistic screening.

INTRODUCTION

Lung cancer is the leading cause of cancer-related mortality.[1,2] Lung cancer screening (LCS) with low-dose computed tomography (LDCT) has been demonstrated in randomized controlled trials to substantially decrease disease-specific mortality.[3,4] As a result, screening programs have been established or are being established in many countries around the world.[2] Current barriers to LCS include slow uptake, low adherence, the time intensive and specialized task of interpreting CT examinations, a high false-positive rate which results in unnecessary anxiety and follow-up investigations, and a mismatch between the population eligible for screening and those diagnosed with lung cancer.[2]

Recent advances in artificial intelligence and machine learning (AI/ML) hold substantial promise to overcome some of these challenges. AI/ML tools commercially available in the United States fall mainly into the category of computer-assisted detection.

This article reviews the current status and future directions of AI/ML in the lung cancer screening workflow (**Fig. 1**). The authors discuss the role of AI/ML for optimizing screening eligibility, radiation dose reduction and image denoising, lung nodule detection, lung nodule classification, and optimizing screening intervals. In addition, the authors outline

[a] Department of Radiology, Stanford University School of Medicine, Stanford, CA, USA; [b] Department of Electrical Engineering and Computer Science, Massachusetts Institute of Technology, Cambridge, MA, USA; [c] Jameel Clinic, Massachusetts Institute of Technology, Cambridge, MA, USA; [d] Department of Medicine, Massachusetts General Hospital, Harvard Medical School, 55 Fruit Street, Boston, MA 02114, USA; [e] Harvard Medical School, Boston, MA, USA; [f] Department of Radiology, Massachusetts General Hospital, 55 Fruit Street, Boston, MA 02114, USA
* Corresponding authors.
E-mail addresses: lvsequist@partners.org (L.V.S.); fintelmann@mgh.harvard.edu (F.J.F.)

Thorac Surg Clin 33 (2023) 401–409
https://doi.org/10.1016/j.thorsurg.2023.03.001
1547-4127/23/© 2023 Elsevier Inc. All rights reserved.

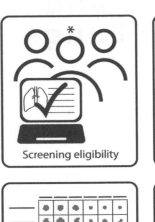
Screening eligibility

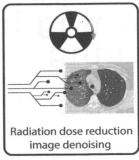
Radiation dose reduction image denoising

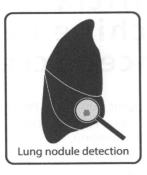
Lung nodule detection

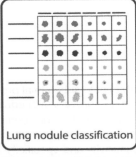
Lung nodule classification

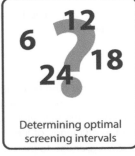
Determining optimal screening intervals

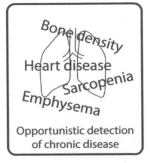
Opportunistic detection of chronic disease

Fig. 1. Applications of artificial intelligence and machine learning across the lung cancer screening workflow.

the role of AI/ML tools to screen for chronic diseases other than lung cancer on LCS LDCT.

DETERMINING SCREENING ELIGIBILITY

In current practice, LCS eligibility is determined using a combination of age and smoking history. In the United States, the 2021 US Preventive Services Task Force (USPSTF) criteria recommend LCS with annual LDCT for individuals aged 50–80 years with a smoking history of at least 20 pack-years.[5] Other jurisdictions such as Canada and the United Kingdom initially apply age and smoking history criteria, followed by risk stratification with the PLCO$_{m2012}$ model or Liverpool Lung Project version 2 (LLP$_{v2}$) model. In this setting, a 6-year lung cancer risk more than 1.51% to 2.50% is required for screening eligibility.[2] AI/ML tools have been used to risk stratify individuals for LCS based on clinical variables and imaging with chest radiography or LDCT.[6–8] Lung cancer risk prediction using AI/ML tools allows for a more comprehensive approach beyond age and smoking history which could help identify individuals most likely to benefit from screening.

Chest radiography may prove to be a useful initial test to risk stratify individuals with low to intermediate lung cancer risk. Compared with LDCT, radiography is less costly and more widely available. Lu and colleagues trained a deep learning model (CXR-LC) to predict up to 12-year lung

cancer risk using age, sex, current smoking status, and chest radiographs as inputs. The model had higher net benefit than the USPSTF 2015 criteria (area under the receiver operating characteristic curve [AUC], 0.755 vs. 0.634; p < 0.001) and similar performance to the PLCO$_{m2012}$ model (CXR-LC AUC of 0.755 vs PLCO$_{m2012}$ AUC of 0.751 in the Prostate, Lung, Colorectal and Ovarian Screening [PLCO] data set and 0.659 vs 0.650 in the National Lung Screening Trial [NLST] data set).[9] In a follow-up study validating the model in a large US hospital system, the 6-year incidence of lung cancer for individuals deemed eligible based on the CXR-LC model but not the USPSTF criteria was 3.3% (121 of 3,703 individuals), which is higher than currently accepted 6-year risk thresholds to define screening eligibility.[6] This suggests that the CXR-LC model may efficiently identify additional patients at high risk of lung cancer who would not otherwise be eligible for lung cancer screening based on USPSTF criteria. Another validation paper showed the model could decrease the number of screening participants while maintaining a similar inclusion rate for incident lung cancer.[10]

As an alternative approach, an ensemble machine learning model of highly parsimonious models was developed by Callender and colleagues[7] with only three variables—age, smoking duration, and pack-years—as inputs. The optimized pipeline was an ensemble of AdaBoost (9.5% pipeline weight), LightGBM (23.8%), logistic regression (42.9%), and linear discriminant analysis (23.8%). The model achieved an AUC of 0.787 for lung cancer prediction in an external validation with higher sensitivity than the USPSTF 2021 criteria at the same specificity.[7] The simplicity of the model helps overcome some of the challenges of current risk prediction models such as $PLCO_{m2012}$ and LLP_{v2} which require clinical variables that are often not readily available.

In contrast to the parsimonious models described above, Gould and colleagues developed a model to predict a future diagnosis of lung cancer based on up to 834 different features from the electronic medical record. The model outperformed a modified version of the $PLCO_{m2012}$ model without a family history of lung cancer (AUC 0.86 vs. 0.79). The 10 most informative features in the model included established risk factors for lung cancer, including age, smoking duration, and pack-years, and novel laboratory predictors including white blood cell count, high-density lipoprotein, and red cell distribution width.[8] Another model which used 1,929 features from ICD-9-CM codes and medication groups achieved a similarly high AUC of 0.90 for prediction of 1-year risk of lung cancer, but was not directly compared with other models.[11]

The distinct epidemiology of lung cancer across certain geographic regions and populations must be carefully considered when developing and deploying AI/ML models for determining screening eligibility. For example, a high proportion of lung cancers in Asia are in females who have never smoked,[12,13] and models trained on data sets in which lung cancer predominantly occurs in individuals with high smoking histories would be expected to miss a substantial number of cancers in those who never smoked. AI/ML tools may perpetuate existing biases and inequalities, particularly if they are not trained with data that represent the population to which the algorithm is applied.[14] Careful selection of training, validation, and testing data sets, which are representative of the population at large, as well as analyses to assess performance in subgroups, are important to ensure that algorithms reduce health care inequities rather than exacerbate them.

RADIATION DOSE REDUCTION AND IMAGE RECONSTRUCTION FOR LOW-DOSE CHEST COMPUTED TOMOGRAPHY

There have been substantial efforts to further reduce the radiation dose associated with LDCT, which may be particularly important considering the expected cumulative life-time radiation exposure for LCS participants. Although ultra-low-dose techniques have been developed, the noise increase associated with radiation dose reduction remains a challenge. Increased image noise makes it more difficult for radiologists to detect small lung nodules. Iterative reconstruction based on raw CT data is an established approach for dose reduction. AI/ML tools which use already reconstructed images as inputs may prove a valid complementary technique to further reduce image noise. Hata and colleagues assessed the effect of combined deep learning-based denoising and iterative reconstruction on ultra-low-dose chest CT. The combined approach of deep learning-based denoising resulted in improved radiologist-rated scores for nodule edge, clarity of small vessels, homogeneity of the normal lung parenchyma, and overall image quality.[15] Another study showed that deep learning image reconstruction reduced image noise, increased lung nodule detection, and improved measurement accuracy on ultra-low-dose chest CT images (0.07 or 0.14 mSv) compared with adaptive statistical iterative reconstruction-V.[16] A phantom study similarly showed that deep learning image reconstruction resulted in higher accuracy compared with model-based iterative reconstruction and hybrid iterative reconstruction for volumetric measurement of artificial ground-glass nodules on ultra-low-dose CT.[17]

LUNG NODULE DETECTION

Lung nodule detection is one of the most established tasks for which AI/ML has been used in the LCS workflow. Traditional image processing techniques for lung nodule detection and segmentation relied primarily on manually engineered algorithms with user-specified parameters. In a typical workflow, a radiologist would first identify a nodule and then provide one or more seeds by clicking inside the nodule, thereby providing a starting point for an algorithm to expand the selection and segment of the nodule from border to border.[18–20] A user could then further refine the segmented region manually.

Using large data sets of natural scenes paired with object and pixel-level annotations, neural networks were applied to object detection and segmentation tasks and have since become the state-of-the-art approach for image analysis.[21–25] In object detection, a neural network is trained to process an image and predict the coordinates of a bounding box that has been previously annotated, as in YOLO[22,23] or Mask-R-CNN.[24] In image segmentation, a neural network is designed to provide predictions at a higher resolution by predicting a label for every pixel (or voxel) in an image, as in U-Net.[25] These models are typically built using convolutional neural networks, or more recently Vision Transformers,[26] to process 2D and 3D imaging data sets along with a classifier that outputs the bounding box or segmentation predictions. Efforts including the Lung Image Database Consortium and Image Database Resource Initiative allowed for the curation of data consisting of chest CTs paired with expert-annotated nodules.[27] This in turn gave rise to the LUNA16 competition for nodule detection where the deep learning methods have since been shown to achieve the state-of-the-art performance.[28–30] For instance, Ardila and colleagues[31] developed a deep learning model for cancer prediction by first automatically extracting pulmonary nodules then classifying these regions of interest to predict the likelihood of lung cancer within 1 and 2 years. In particular, a Mask-R-CNN model was trained on LUNA16 to obtain lung segmentation predictions, and a second model based on RetinaNet was used to obtain the bounding boxes of individual nodules.[31]

The reported sensitivity and specificity of AI/ML algorithms for lung nodule detection range from 75% to 100% and 83% to 96%, respectively.[29] Although one of the challenges of AI/ML tools has historically been a high false-positive rate, a deep learning algorithm recently showed higher sensitivity for lung nodule detection than double reading, with a false-positive rate of only one nodule per scan.[32] Such tools may also reduce interpretation time, with one study showing a 26% reduction in interpretation time when using a combined pulmonary vessel image-suppressed function and computer-aided detection system.[33] Commercially available software also allows for direct comparison of nodules between examinations, which may further improve interpretation efficiency.

LUNG NODULE CLASSIFICATION AND LUNG CANCER RISK PREDICTION

Imaging-based methods for lung cancer prediction include those that classify nodules based on manually defined or learned features as well as methods that consider the entire LDCT volume. Focusing on indeterminate pulmonary nodules, Hawkins and colleagues[34] used a combination of 219 image features (such as nodule size and texture) from baseline screening LDCT acquired during the NLST to predict subsequent cancer development and achieved an AUC of 0.83 and 0.75 for 1- and 2-year predictions, respectively. On the other hand, Huang and colleagues[35] used nodule and non-nodule features to predict lung cancer incidence up to 3 years

after the last screening LDCT for participants of the PanCan study, with AUCs ranging from 0.899 to -0.968.

On the other hand, a deep learning model called Sybil (**Fig. 2**)[36] was developed to predict lung cancer risk up to 6 years based on a single LCS LDCT and was validated on data from the NLST as well as external data from Massachusetts General Hospital and Chang Gung Memorial Hospital in Taiwan. The advantages of Sybil include that the code is publicly accessible and that the model does not require any human input. In addition, Sybil does not only consider nodules but evaluates risk based on the entire 3D image stack. On the other hand, the pipeline developed by Ardila and colleagues[31] combines nodule detection with nodule classification and cancer detection by first learning to extract individual lesions and then using the regions of interest along with the full low-dose CT volume to predict 1- and 2-year cancer development, achieving ROC-AUCs of 0.944 and 0.873, respectively, on a held out subset of the NLST.

Similarly, LungNet[37] was developed as a convolutional neural network that learns directly to classify nodules and predict survival of patients with non-small cell lung cancer from preprocessed voxels of extracted lung lesions.

As texture and wavelet features used for lung nodule classification can be substantially affected by the reconstruction kernel, using deep learning to convert images to standardized kernels may improve generalizability of AI/ML lung nodule classifiers across scanners, vendors, and institutions. Choe and colleagues[38] found that image conversion using a convolutional neural network improved the reproducibility of radiomic features for pulmonary nodules or masses, with the concordance correlation coefficient improving from 0.38 to 0.84 for kernel-converted images.

The AI/ML algorithms for lung nodule stratification are now commercially available and have received clearance by the US Food and Drug Administration and Health Canada as well as the CE marking by the European Union. Compared with Lung-RADS version 1.1, the standardized clinical reporting system for LCS LDCT in the United States, one algorithm demonstrated increased sensitivity and specificity for classification of LCS studies.[39] When analyzing preceding scans of malignant nodules 2 years before a confirmed diagnosis of lung cancer, 42% of these nodules were deemed to be high risk, which could help establish a diagnosis of lung cancer 1 year earlier and potentially at an earlier stage.[39]

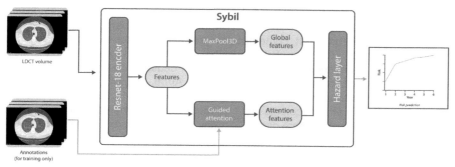

Fig. 2. Architecture of an end-to-end deep learning algorithm for lung cancer risk prediction. Features from the low-dose CT volume are extracted using a pretrained 3D Resnet-18 encoder and subsequently used to compute a global feature vector through a Max Pooling layer. Lung nodules which are annotated with bounding boxes are used as inputs to an attention-guided pooling layer to guide the model's attention during training. The resulting vectors are concatenated and passed through a hazard layer, with the output of cumulative probability of developing lung cancer. (*Adapted from* Mikhael PG, Wohlwend J, Yala A, et al. Sybil: A Validated Deep Learning Model to Predict Future Lung Cancer Risk From a Single Low-Dose Chest Computed Tomography J Clin Oncol. 2023 Apr 20;41(12):2191-2200. doi: 10.1200/JCO.22.01345. Epub 2023 Jan 12.)

Increased specificity in terms of classification of screen-detected lung nodules as benign and potentially malignant by AI/ML tools may reduce patient anxiety as well as the number of follow-up investigations, including chest CT, PET/CT, and biopsies. One study assessed the cost impact of combining Lung-RADS with an end-to-end AI/ML tool[31] to "upgrade" or "downgrade" Lung-RADS categories based on malignancy risk scores.[40] Cost-savings were estimated to be at least $72 per patient screened using the AI-informed management compared with Lung-RADS alone.[40] AI/ML tools could increase the cost-effectiveness of lung cancer screening, potentially enabling expanded eligibility for lung cancer screening and allowing countries with limited resources to implement efficient LCS programs. Improved characterization through AI/ML tools could also help replace subspecialty thoracic imaging expertise when and where such expertise is unavailable.

PERSONALIZED SCREENING INTERVALS

Most current LCS guidelines, including from the USPSTF, recommend annual screening with LDCT.[5] However, there is substantial interest in defining individuals for whom biannual screening may be sufficient. The goal is to minimize the total number of CT scans without increasing morbidity and mortality potentially associated with a delayed cancer diagnosis.

Various multivariable regression models have been developed to predict future lung cancer risk and modify screening intervals. For example, Robbins and colleagues[41] combined clinical risk factors and LDCT-based features to calculate

1- and 2-year cancer risk and demonstrated how such predictions could be used to better modulate patient screening intervals. The $PLCO_{m2012}$ model was extended to directly incorporate screening results through Lung-RADS scores assigned by radiologists ($PLCO_{m2012results}$).[42] Developed on the data from the NLST, the $PLCO_{2012results}$ model used the screening outcomes of all three rounds performed in the trial to predict cancer risk 1 to 4 years following the last examination. The model was used to identify participants who should continue to undergo annual screening, and participants for whom the screening interval could be safely extended to 2 years.[42]

Open access end-to-end AI/ML risk prediction algorithms without the need for human input or annotation such as Sybil developed by Mikhael and colleagues[36] may be an effective way to stratify patients into high- and low-risk categories for developing an interval cancer over the next 2 years and enable biannual screening. Higher risk individuals would continue with annual screening or potentially even shorter interval LDCT. Direct comparison to non-AI/ML regression models (eg, $PLCO_{m2012results}$) will be helpful to determine the additional value of these algorithms. Further work will also be required to define risk thresholds for each time interval.

OPPORTUNISTIC SCREENING

Assessing for chronic diseases beyond lung cancer on screening LDCT may be a substantial opportunity to improve population health. Cardiovascular disease, body composition analysis including bone mineral density, and emphysema are some of the most promising applications for AI/ML in this setting.

Cardiovascular disease is the most common cause of mortality among LCS populations, exceeding mortality from lung cancer.[3,4] The accurate prediction of cardiovascular risk at the time of LCS is an important opportunity to identify patients who may benefit from pharmacologic and non-pharmacologic intervention to reduce cardiovascular risk, and quantifying risk based on imaging may promote patient adherence to such therapies. Deep learning models can quantify coronary artery calcium on routine non-ECG-gated chest LCS LDCT scans.

Eng and colleagues[43] trained a convolutional neural network to perform (1) segmentation of calcium lesions that contribute to the Agatston score and (2) categorization of each calcium lesion as belonging to the left main, left anterior descending, left circumflex, or right coronary arteries. For routine non-gated chest CTs, an additional step was performed with summary vectors of segmentation outputs used as inputs to a gradient-boosted decision tree classifier. For non-gated chest CTs, the model achieved sensitivities of 71% to 94% and positive predictive values of 88% to 100% for coronary artery calcium scores ≥100 across validation cohorts.[43]

Other studies have similarly shown promising results for deep learning quantification of coronary calcium from non-gated chest CT examinations. An algorithm consisting of two convolutional neural networks achieved intraclass correlation coefficients of 0.97 (95% confidence interval [CI]: 0.96, 0.97) between automatically and manually obtained scores when applied to ECG-gated coronary artery calcium CT examinations, and 0.90 (95% CI: 0.88, 0.92) when applied to non-gated chest CT.[44] A study assessing 5-year cardiovascular disease mortality prediction in the NLST cohort showed that a model incorporating deep learning-quantified arterial calcification—including coronary artery calcification, thoracic aorta calcification, and aortic and mitral valve calcification—from LDCT may have better predictive ability than a model with self-reported participant characteristics alone (C-statistic of 0.76; 95% CI: 0.71–0.80 vs. 0.69; 95% CI: 0.64–0.74), although this difference was not statistically significant.[45]

There is increasing evidence demonstrating the association between adipose tissue and cardiovascular disease.[46,47] AI/ML tools which automate adipose tissue quantification on chest CT may augment traditional cardiovascular risk prediction models.[48] Automated quantification of muscle mass can diagnose sarcopenia on chest CT[48]—a condition that has been associated with increased mortality in LCS participants.[49]

Vertebral fractures and bone mineral density have been shown to be independently associated with all-cause mortality among LCS participants.[50] Using AI/ML to provide information about osteopenia and identify individuals who may benefit from preventive therapy may be another opportunity to further increase the value of lung cancer screening. The current state-of-the-art approaches first use a convolutional neural network to segment and label the vertebral bodies, followed by a second neural network or linear function to determine bone mineral density.[51,52] AI/ML algorithms have also been developed to quantify emphysema on low-dose chest CT examinations,[53–55] which may help inform screening selection criteria (with consideration given to emphysema as a risk factor for lung cancer as well as a competing cause of death), screening intervals, and preventive interventions such as smoking cessation.[2]

LIMITATIONS

Machine learning is fundamentally limited by the quality of the annotated data sets available to train and evaluate models.[56] Image data sets available from the NLST highlight the advantages of providing the AI/ML research community with open access to large annotated clinical data sets. Yet, vast quantities of data in hospitals and other institutions remain unstructured and beyond the reach of the AI/ML research community. In particular, there is an important need for data sets with increased population diversity. The democratization of access to data can further enhance the robustness of AI/ML models and improve adoption, paving the way for improved outcomes for patients.

SUMMARY

Continued advances in AI/ML hold significant promise to further increase the efficiency of lung cancer screening in a variety of global settings, potentially increasing the number of individuals who may benefit from screening and improving equity in LCS. The potential for AI/ML to assess for other chronic diseases on CT presents an additional opportunity to improve population health and may further increase the value of lung cancer screening. Important future steps include implementation studies examining the optimal clinical use of these novel tools and further characterization of their strengths and limitations in real-world applications.

CLINICS CARE POINTS

- When considering the clinical implementation of an artificial intelligence (AI) tool for lung cancer screening, ensure the AI tool was trained on data reflecting the population it is being used for, has been externally validated, and has regulatory approval.

- Seek AI tools that allow visual confirmation of results (verifiable AI).

- Ensure the AI tool does not send patient data to a third party unless you have clearance to use such a tool.

- Recognize that AI tools may identify patients who are at high risk for lung cancer and who may not meet the US Preventive Services Task Force eligibility criteria for lung cancer screening; such individuals may not qualify for reimbursement.

- Consider creating care coordination pathways that allow health systems to effectively act on AI-detected opportunistic findings such as coronary artery calcification, sarcopenia, and osteoporosis.

DISCLOSURES

R. Barzilay: Leadership: Dewpoint Therapeutics. Consulting or Advisory Role: J&J, Amgen, Outcomes4Me, Immunai, Firmenich. Travel, Accommodations, Expenses: J&J, Firmenich. L.V. Sequist: Research funding: AstraZeneca, Novartis, Genentech, Delfi. Consulting: Janssen, Pfizer, Takeda. F.J. Fintelmann: Salary support from the William M Wood Foundation for unrelated research. Consulting: Pfizer. The other authors declare no relevant conflict of interest.

REFERENCES

1. Sung H, Ferlay J, Siegel RL, et al. Global cancer statistics 2020: GLOBOCAN estimates of incidence and mortality worldwide for 36 cancers in 185 countries. CA Cancer J Clin 2021;71(3):209–49.

2. Adams SJ, Stone E, Baldwin DR, et al. Lung cancer screening. Lancet 2023;401(10374):390–408.

3. National Lung Screening Trial Research Team, Aberle DR, Adams AM, et al. Reduced lung-cancer mortality with low-dose computed tomographic screening. N Engl J Med 2011;365(5):395–409.

4. de Koning HJ, Van Der Aalst CM, De Jong PA, et al. Reduced lung-cancer mortality with volume CT screening in a randomized trial. N Engl J Med 2020;382(6):503–13.

5. US Preventive Services Task Force, Krist AH, Davidson KW, et al. Screening for lung cancer: US preventive services task force recommendation statement. JAMA 2021;325(10):962–70.

6. Raghu VK, Walia AS, Zinzuwadia AN, et al. Validation of a deep learning-based model to predict lung cancer risk using chest radiographs and electronic medical record data. JAMA Netw Open 2022;5(12):e2248793.

7. Callender T, Imrie F, Cebere B, et al. Assessing eligibility for lung cancer screening: parsimonious multi-country ensemble machine learning models for lung cancer prediction. medRxiv 2023;1–26.

8. Gould MK, Huang BZ, Tammemagi MC, et al. Machine learning for early lung cancer identification using routine clinical and laboratory data. Am J Respir Crit Care Med 2021;204(4):445–53.

9. Lu MT, Raghu VK, Mayrhofer T, et al. Deep learning using chest radiographs to identify high-risk smokers for lung cancer screening computed tomography: development and validation of a prediction model. Ann Intern Med 2020;173(9):704–13.

10. Lee JH, Lee D, Lu MT, et al. Deep learning to optimize candidate selection for lung cancer CT screening: advancing the 2021 USPSTF recommendations. Radiology 2022;305(1):209–18.

11. Yeh MCH, Wang YH, Yang HC, et al. Artificial intelligence‖based prediction of lung cancer risk using nonimaging electronic medical records: Deep learning approach. J Med Internet Res 2021;23(8):1–13.

12. Sun S, Schiller JH, Gazdar AF. Lung cancer in never smokers - a different disease. Nat Rev Cancer 2007;7(10):778–90.

13. Lam S. Lung cancer screening in never-smokers. J Thorac Oncol 2019;14(3):336–7.

14. Celi LA, Cellini J, Charpignon M-L, et al. Sources of bias in artificial intelligence that perpetuate healthcare disparities—A global review. PLOS Digit Heal 2022;1(3):e0000022.

15. Hata A, Yanagawa M, Yoshida Y, et al. Combination of deep learning–based denoising and iterative reconstruction for ultra-low-dose CT of the chest: image quality and Lung-RADS evaluation. Am J Roentgenol 2020;(215):1321–8.

16. Jiang B, Li N, Shi X, et al. Deep learning reconstruction shows better lung nodule detection for ultra–low-dose chest CT. Radiology 2022;303(1):202–12.

17. Mikayama R, Shirasaka T, Kojima T, et al. Deep-learning reconstruction for ultra-low-dose lung CT: volumetric measurement accuracy and reproducibility of artificial ground-glass nodules in a phantom study. Br J Radiol 2022;95(1130). https://doi.org/10.1259/bjr.20210915.

18. Carmo D, Ribeiro J, Dertkigil S, et al. A systematic review of automated segmentation methods and

public datasets for the lung and its lobes and findings on computed tomography images. Yearb Med Inform 2022;31(1):277–95.

19. Maldonado F, Boland JM, Raghunath S, et al. Noninvasive characterization of the histopathologic features of pulmonary nodules of the lung adenocarcinoma spectrum using computer-aided nodule assessment and risk yield (CANARY) - A pilot study. J Thorac Oncol 2013;8(4):452–60.

20. Gu Y, Kumar V, Hall LO, et al. Automated delineation of lung tumors from CT images using a single click ensemble segmentation approach. Pattern Recognit 2013;46(3):692–702.

21. Girshick R. Fast R-CNN. arXiv. 2015. https://doi.org/10.48550/arXiv.1504.08083.

22. Redmon J, Divvala S, Girshick R, et al. You only look once: unified, real-time object detection, *arXiv*, 2016. https://doi.org/10.48550/arXiv.1506.02640.

23. Ge Z, Liu S, Wang F, et al. YOLOX: exceeding YOLO Series in 2021. arXiv 2021;. https://doi.org/10.48550/arXiv.2107.08430.

24. He K, Gkioxari G, Piotr D, et al. MaskR-CNN. arXiv 2018;. https://doi.org/10.48550/arXiv.1703.06870.

25. Ronneberger O, Fischer P, and Brox T. U-Net: Convolutional Networks for Biomedical Image Segmentation, *arXiv*, 2015. https://doi.org/10.48550/arXiv.1505.04597.

26. Liu Z, Lin Y, Cao Y, et al. Swin Transformer: Hierarchical Vision Transformer using Shifted Windows, *arXiv*, 2021. https://doi.org/10.48550/arXiv.2103.14030.

27. Armato SG, McLennan G, Bidaut L, et al. The Lung Image Database Consortium (LIDC) and Image Database Resource Initiative (IDRI): A completed reference database of lung nodules on CT scans. Med Phys 2011;38(2):915–31.

28. Setio AAA, Traverso A, de Bel T, et al. Validation, comparison, and combination of algorithms for automatic detection of pulmonary nodules in computed tomography images: the LUNA16 challenge. Med Image Anal 2017;42:1–13.

29. Li D, Vilmun BM, Carlsen JF, et al. The performance of deep learning algorithms on automatic pulmonary nodule detection and classification tested on different datasets that are not derived from LIDC-IDRI: a systematic review. Diagnostics 2019;9(4):207.

30. Pehrson LM, Nielsen MB, Lauridsen CA. Automatic pulmonary nodule detection applying deep learning or machine learning algorithms to the LIDC-IDRI database: a systematic review. Diagnostics 2019; 9(29):1–11.

31. Ardila D, Kiraly AP, Bharadwaj S, et al. End-to-end lung cancer screening with three-dimensional deep learning on low-dose chest computed tomography. Nat Med 2019;25(6):954–61.

32. Cui X, Zheng S, Heuvelmans MA, et al. Performance of a deep learning-based lung nodule detection

system as an alternative reader in a Chinese lung cancer screening program. Eur J Radiol 2022;146: 110068.

33. Lo SCB, Freedman MT, Gillis LB, et al. Computeraided detection of lung nodules on CT with a computerized pulmonary vessel suppressed function. Am J Roentgenol 2018;210(3):480–8.

34. Hawkins S, Wang H, Liu Y, et al. Predicting malignant nodules from screening CT scans. J Thorac Oncol 2016;11(12):2120–8.

35. Huang P, Lin CT, Li Y, et al. Prediction of lung cancer risk at follow-up screening with low-dose CT: a training and validation study of a deep learning method. Lancet Digit Heal 2019;1(7):e353–62.

36. Mikhael PPG, Wohlwend J, Yala A, et al. Sybil: a validated deep learning model to predict future lung cancer risk from a single low-dose chest computed tomography. J Clin Oncol 2023;41(12):2191–200.

37. Mukherjee P, Zhou M, Lee E, et al. A shallow convolutional neural network predicts prognosis of lung cancer patients in multi-institutional computed tomography image datasets. Nat Mach Intell 2020; 2(5):274–82.

38. Choe J, Lee SM, Do KH, et al. Deep learning–based image conversion of CT reconstruction kernels improves radiomics reproducibility for pulmonary nodules or masses. Radiology 2019;292(2):365–73.

39. Adams SJ, Madtes DK, Burbridge B, et al. Clinical impact and generalizability of a computer-assisted diagnostic tool to risk-stratify lung nodules with CT. J Am Coll Radiol 2023;20:232–42.

40. Adams SJ, Mondal P, Penz E, et al. Development and cost analysis of a lung nodule management strategy combining artificial intelligence and Lung-RADS for baseline lung cancer screening. J Am Coll Radiol 2021;18(5):741–51.

41. Robbins HA, Cheung LC, Chaturvedi AK, et al. Management of lung cancer screening results based on individual prediction of current and future lung cancer risks. J Thorac Oncol 2022;17(2):252–63.

42. Tammemägi MC, Ten Haaf K, Toumazis I, et al. Development and validation of a multivariable lung cancer risk prediction model that includes lowdose computed tomography screening results: a secondary analysis of data from the National Lung Screening Trial. JAMA Netw Open 2019;2(3): e190204.

43. Eng D, Chute C, Khandwala N, et al. Automated coronary calcium scoring using deep learning with multicenter external validation. npj Digit Med 2021; 4(1). https://doi.org/10.1038/s41746-021-00460-1.

44. van Velzen SGM, Lessmann N, Velthuis BK, et al. Deep learning for automatic calcium scoring in CT: validation using multiple cardiac CT and chest CT protocols. Radiology 2020;295(1):66–79.

45. de Vos BD, Lessmann N, de Jong PA, et al. Deep learning–quantified calcium scores for automatic

cardiovascular mortality prediction at lung screening low-dose CT. Radiol Cardiothorac Imaging 2021;3(2). https://doi.org/10.1148/ryct. 2021190219.

46. Maurovich-Horvat P, Kallianos K, Engel LC, et al. Relationship of thoracic fat depots with coronary atherosclerosis and circulating inflammatory biomarkers. Obesity 2015;23(6):1178–84.

47. Akawi N, Checa A, Antonopoulos AS, et al. Fat-secreted ceramides regulate vascular redox state and influence outcomes in patients with cardiovascular disease. J Am Coll Cardiol 2021;77(20): 2494–513.

48. Bridge CP, Best TD, Wrobel MM, et al. A fully automated deep learning pipeline for multi-vertebral level quantification and characterization of muscle and adipose tissue on chest CT scans. Radiol Artif Intell 2022;4(1):1–7.

49. Lenchik L, Barnard R, Boutin RD, et al. Automated muscle measurement on chest CT predicts all-cause mortality in older adults from the National Lung Screening Trial. Journals Gerontol - Ser A Biol Sci Med Sci. 2021;76(2):277–85.

50. Buckens CF, van der Graaf Y, Verkooijen HM, et al. Osteoporosis markers on low-dose lung cancer screening chest computed tomography scans predict all-cause mortality. Eur Radiol 2015;25(1):132–9.

51. Fang Y, Li W, Chen X, et al. Opportunistic osteoporosis screening in multi-detector CT images using deep convolutional neural networks. Eur Radiol 2021;31(4):1831–42.

52. Pan Y, Shi D, Wang H, et al. Automatic opportunistic osteoporosis screening using low-dose chest computed tomography scans obtained for lung cancer screening. Eur Radiol 2020;30(7):4107–16.

53. Yeom JA, Kim KU, Hwang M, et al. Emphysema quantification using ultra-low-dose chest CT: efficacy of deep learning-based image reconstruction. Med 2022;58(7):1–12.

54. Jin H, Heo C, Kim JH. Deep learning-enabled accurate normalization of reconstruction kernel effects on emphysema quantification in low-dose CT. Phys Med Biol 2019;64(13). https://doi.org/10.1088/1361-6560/ab28a1.

55. Tanabe N, Kaji S, Shima H, et al. Kernel conversion for robust quantitative measurements of archived chest computed tomography using deep learning-based image-to-image translation. Front Artif Intell 2022;4(January):1–12.

56. Chen X, Wang X, Zhang K, et al. Recent advances and clinical applications of deep learning in medical image analysis. Med Image Anal 2022;79:102444.

Liquid Biopsy as an Adjunct to Lung Screening Imaging

Nathaniel Deboever, MD[a], Edwin J. Ostrin, MD, PhD[b], Mara B. Antonoff, MD[a],*

KEYWORDS

- Lung cancer screening • Liquid biopsy • Low-dose computed tomography scan
- Disease monitoring

KEY POINTS

- Lung cancer screening has great potential in reducing cancer-related deaths.
- Low-dose computed tomography (LDCT) is currently used as the main screening modality; however, utilization is low and rate of false positives is high.
- Liquid biopsy can personalize risk stratification in lung cancer screening.
- A combination of LDCT and liquid biopsy may improve uptake and rate of false positives associated with the current screening paradigm.

CURRENT STATE OF LUNG CANCER SCREENING

Benefits of Lung Cancer Screening

Despite recent advances in strategies for management, lung cancer remains the leading cause of cancer-related death, affecting people worldwide as the second most common malignancy.[1,2] An underlying cause of its high mortality associated is delayed diagnoses with the most cases being diagnosed as advanced disease.[3–6] An obvious solution to this challenge is the implementation of a robust screening system. In 2011, the National Lung Screening Trial (NLST) showed that low-dose computed tomography (LDCT) can reduce lung cancer mortality by 20% in high-risk individuals, which was attributable to the earlier detection of disease.[7–9] In 2013, the US Preventive Services Task Force (USPSTF) endorsed annual LDCT for high-risk individuals, defined as men and women aged 55 to 74 years with a 30-pack-year smoking history, who were either currently smoking or who had quit within the prior 15 years.[10] This recommendation was ultimately supported by Centers for Medicare and Medicaid Services (CMS).[11] Subsequently, these criteria were broadened in 2021 to individuals aged ≥ 50 years and with ≥ 20-pack-year smoking history based on modeling showing predicted benefit.[12] In a real-world evaluation, Khouzam and colleagues showed that adherence to these public health interventions led to stage-shifting toward earlier stage lung cancers. Furthermore, the investigators showed that screening was associated with a 14.2 per 100,000 persons absolute reduction in the incidence of advanced-stage lung cancer.[13] Screening for lung cancer can have a profound effect on public health by capturing early disease and enabling patients to receive curative therapy.

Challenges with Lung Cancer Screening Utilization

Unfortunately, screening utilization in the United States has been underwhelming with only 6% of eligible patients receiving the recommended

---

[a] Department of Thoracic and Cardiovascular Surgery, University of Texas MD Anderson Cancer Center, 1515 Holcombe Boulevard, Houston, TX 77030, USA; [b] Department of General Internal Medicine, Pulmonary Medicine, University of Texas MD Anderson Cancer Center, 1515 Holcombe Boulevard, Houston, TX 77030, USA
* Corresponding author. 1400 Pressler Street Unit 1489, Houston, TX.
E-mail address: MBAntonoff@MDAnderson.org

Thorac Surg Clin 33 (2023) 411–419
https://doi.org/10.1016/j.thorsurg.2023.04.004
1547-4127/23/© 2023 Elsevier Inc. All rights reserved.

annual LDCT in 2015.[1] Implementation failed to increase over time, with 5.8% reported in 2021 across the United States,[14] and 16.3% in states that have rolled out statewide screening programs.[15] As these numbers were reported, broadened criteria have increased eligibility from 8 to 14 million individuals in the United States. Complicating the challenges of low screening rates, follow-up after LDCT is also poor.[16] This challenge may be due to geographic differences across the United States. For example, smoking habits are increased in rural areas, which may have reduced access to lung cancer screening programs.[17] Definition and documentation of smoking history may impact likelihood of lung cancer screening recommendations,[18] particularly in this population. In addition, there is difference in access to lung cancer diagnosis for rural patients.[19] Although similar screening uptake between rural and urban settings has been reported,[20] higher incidence of lung cancer in rural areas should warrant increased resource allocation.[21] This phenomenon has led to rural and suburban residents having higher rates of unstaged disease,[22] in addition to lower rates of adequate treatment of lung cancer.[23] Moreover, there may be social and psychological barriers to lung cancer screening, including a decreased ability to attend LDCT facilities secondary to location or family support to attend screening[24] or false beliefs regarding effect of screening.[25] Last, a particular concern in the community is postoperative morbidity and mortality in the event of a positive screen and lung cancer diagnosis.[26]

Given the known challenges associated with present screening adoption, biomarker tests carry potential for an important role to augment use of lung cancer screening by improving efficacy, optimizing efficiency, and alleviating concerns.

LIQUID BIOPSY AND PERIPHERAL BIOMARKERS FOR LUNG CANCER SCREENING

Peripheral blood markers are increasingly used for prognostication of disease. This approach is also used in the diagnosis of cancer and relies on the recognition of circulating biomarkers. These noninvasive tests can complement current screening modalities by focusing on multiple tumor-derived components, such as circulating cell-free DNA (cfDNA) or microRNA (miRNA) originating from the tumor,[27] proteins, metabolites, tumor-educated platelets (TEPs), or tumor-derived exosomes.[28] Biomarkers can serve to refine risk, but, in contrast, may not necessarily depend on tumor components. However, although the development of an early diagnostic biomarker is urgently needed, adequate sensitivity and specificity are paramount to its success in supplementing current lung cancer screening protocols. Detection of tumor-derived components has typically been limited by low sensitivity in the early detection setting, where tumor burden may be low.[29–32] Elevated false negative tests will delay diagnosis, and elevated false-positive tests will lead to unnecessary procedures, systemic burden, and increased patient worry.

Modalities for Blood-Based Assays

cfDNA, including circulating tumor DNA (ctDNA), can be measured to assess the presence of cancer with the added benefit of providing insight on tumor-specific characteristics, such as genetic and epigenetic alterations.[33] Broadly, ctDNA measurements can be meaningful in later stage ($\geq$T2b) lung cancer, whereas cfDNA can provide insights in earlier stage ($\leq$T1b) cancers.[34,35] This is believed to be secondary to the metabolic tumor volume and histopathology.[34] This modality is highly sensitive via pathologic complete response (PCR) and next-generation sequencing (NGS)[28] and can be detected up to 6 to 12 months before radiographic cancer diagnosis[36] and up to 5.2 months before radiographic evidence of progression in patients with managed lung cancer.[37]

miRNA can be obtained from various body fluids, and commercial kits are available; however, its use as a biomarker is associated with high variability.[28] In preliminary exploratory studies, miRNA has showed potential as an adjunct to LDCT with a dose–response relationship[27]; however, it is currently not validated, nor is it specific enough to differentiate cancer types.[38] The bioMILD randomized trial examined the efficacy of incorporating a miRNA signature classifier (MSC) with LDCT for lung cancer screening among eligible patients in Italy.[39] The results showed that a positive MSC was linked to a higher incidence of lung cancer after 4 years, as evidenced by a hazard ratio (HR) of 2.02 (95% confidence interval [CI]: 1.40 to 2.90, p: <0.001). However, the use of MSC did not improve its predictability when LDCT results were negative (HR: 1.51, 95CIL 0.69–3.32, $P = .30$). It is conceivable that the sample size of this subgroup was insufficient to detect a meaningful difference. In contrast, for patients with positive LDCT results, a positive MSC was associated with increased lung cancer incidence ($P < .001$). TEPs are a dynamic biomarker due to the short lifespan of platelets, which is characterized by intraplatelet RNA splicing, thought to be secondary to cancer.[40] The role of TEPs in carcinogenesis continues to be investigated and may relate to angiogenesis or mechanical immunoprotection.[28]

However, one limitation of this biomarker as a liquid biopsy adjunct to LDCT is its potential vulnerability to confounding from anticoagulants, cancer therapy, and inflammatory diseases.[41]

Tumor-derived exosomes contain various types of biomarkers, including proteins and nucleic acids. Exosomes may correlate with carcinogenesis due to their role in immune response regulation and angiogenesis[42] or cell-to-cell communication.[43,44] This biomarker may be available from various body fluids and also has potential as a liquid biomarker for lung cancer,[44] following standardization of extraction and validation[45] even in early stage cancer.[46]

Circulating tumor cells can provide molecular characterization of the primary tumor and metastases[47] and have a role in prognostication of disease.[28] These can be used in early-stage lung cancer.[48]

Metabolomic profiling is another biomarker that may be helpful as we endeavor to increase accuracy of screening protocols. This modality assesses endogenous metabolites produced by cancer cells, which are different from those produced by benign cells.[49] As such, metabolomic profiling can report on the dynamic aspect of function and cancer tissue.[50]

Autoantibodies and protein-based biomarkers (oncoproteomics) evaluate immune system modeling and protein modifications[49] secondary to oncogenesis. Considering the early humoral immune response to tumor antigens, autoantibodies are used as an early detection marker.[50] As the protein-based biomarkers constitute the downstream effects of nucleic-acid modifications, their assessments can provide insight on the oncologic proteome or its posttranslational modification.[51] These tests are currently used for diagnosis as well as disease monitoring.[50] Although the assessment of the proteome can be exploratory, antibody arrays are more sensitive secondary to their ability for serologic profiling.[51] Antibody arrays can be combined into comprehensive panels, capable of achieving reasonable sensitivities and specificities.[52]

Currently Available Tests

Currently, there are a few biomarkers that have undergone external validation (**Table 1**).

NODIFY-LUNG (Nodify Lung Nodule Risk Management, Biodesix, Boulder, CO, USA) is a composite panel (Nodify CDT and Nodify XL2, Biodesix, Boulder, CO, USA) aimed to identify likely malignant indeterminate pulmonary nodules. This test can assist with nodule stratification. Nodify CDT is a seven-autoantibody panel aimed to identify high-risk individuals for LDCT. The test

Table 1
Currently available lung cancer screening adjunct biomarkers

Name	Modality	Main Strategy	Strengths	Drawbacks from Any Tests
NODIFY-LUNG	Composite autoantibody (NodifyCDT and Nodify XL2)	Stratify indeterminate pulmonary nodules	Validated across separate case-control studies 89% specificity in at risk population	• Rates of false positives associated with overdiagnosis • Rates of false negatives associated with delayed diagnoses • Markers (such as GRAIL) may require highly sensitive processing • High sensitivity (GRAIL) in advanced disease may not translate to high sensitivity in early-stage disease
Percepta	Genomic classifier combined with next-generation RNA transcriptome sequencing	Stratify potentially nondiagnostic bronchoscopy results	Informs decision-making in low- and intermediate-risk lung nodules	
GRAIL	DNA methylation assay	Multi-cancer signal detection	Overall specificity of 99.5% in advanced disease	
DELFI	DNA fragmentomics assay	Assess gene-regulation	Overall specificity over 95% in solid cancers	

Abbreviations: ctDNA, circulating tumor DNA; cfDNA, cell-free DNA.

(previously called EarlyCDT-Lung, Oncimmune, Nottingham, UK) has been validated in multiple separate case-control studies[53-55] as well as in routine clinical practice where a positive result was associated with a 5.4-fold increase in lung cancer incidence[56] and was found to have a specificity of 89% in at-risk populations.[57] This test has provided meaningful results in both early- and late-stage disease across histopathologies.[58] Nodify XL2 (Biodesix, Boulder, CO, USA) is a mass spectrometry based 13-protein proteomic panel, achieving a 90% negative predictive value for benign nodules.[59] These results were further used to demonstrate the potential sparing of 31.8% subjects from invasive procedures.[60]

The Percepta genomic classifier is a tool capable to risk stratify bronchoscopy results that may otherwise be nondiagnostic by using cytologic brushings obtained from the mainstem bronchi before lesion sampling.[61] This classifier can inform decision-making by reclassifying risk and upgrading or down-grading risk in patients who otherwise have low- and intermediate-risk lung nodules.[62] A version of Percepta using nasal brushings is currently under development.

The GRAIL DNA methylation assay is a blood-based biomarker capable to detect shared multi-cancer signals, by evaluating methylation patterns of cfDNA[63,64] (18–19). This method was initially validated in a case-control study using the Circulating Cell-free Genome Atlas (17), in which it yielded an overall specificity of 99.5%.[65]

The "DNA Evaluation of Fragments for Early Interception" (DELFI) fragmentomics assay is a biomarker based on the evaluation of patterns in the fragmentation of cfDNA to assess gene

regulatory maps.[66,67] As such, this approach has yielded a specificity beyond 95% in 236 patients with breast, colorectal, lung, ovarian, pancreatic, gastric, or bile duct cancer.[68]

Another promising biomarker is a four-marker protein panel (4MP), consisting of precursors of surfactant protein B, cancer antigen 125, carcinoembryonic antigen, and cytokeratin-19. In combination with the lung cancer risk prediction model prostate lung colorectal ovarian model 2012 ($PLCO_{m2012}$),[69] 4MP was able to yield a risk assessment that was superior to the USPSTF criteria from 2021.[70] It has also been demonstrated to aid in distinguishing benign from malignant indeterminate nodules.[71]

ADVANCES IN BLOOD-BASED ASSAYS FOR LUNG CANCER

Looking to the future, the use of a blood-based adjunct to LDCT for lung cancer screening could be used in two different use cases: (1) to personalize the eligibility criteria for radiographic screening and (2) to stratify patients for therapy following LDCT (**Fig. 1**).

Pre-Imaging Assay

Increasing eligibility and access to lung cancer screening is urgently needed, as failure to do so continues to expand health care disparities.[72-74] A noninvasive, non-radiographic screening test as an adjunct to LDCT may enhance the risk assessment of otherwise currently ineligible populations, which inequitably includes women and racial minorities.[75] A pre-imaging blood-based adjunct to LDCT may alleviate potential system- and patient-level barriers

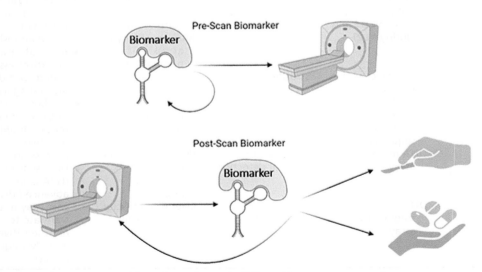

Fig. 1. Two pathways to using biomarker adjuncts in CT-based lung cancer screening.

to lung cancer screening. As LDCT uptake continues to increase following public health interventions, health care systems may be overburdened, specifically in lung screening facility geographic deserts.[76] A non-radiographic approach may help identify subjects who most warrant LDCT screening and further encourage these individuals to travel to a lung screening facility. In addition, a blood-based adjunct to LDCT may also mitigate patient-level barriers such as unjustified reservations relating to radiation exposure[77] from the current screening paradigm.

Importantly, a synergistic complement to the current radiographic screening system would provide a personalized assessment of individuals who are defined as low risk by current guidelines, such as heavy smokers who quit more than 15 years before screening or light ongoing smokers.

Post-Imaging Assay

Increasing eligibility for lung cancer screening may result in less mortality and increased life years gained[78]; however, false positives may increase, leading to unnecessary invasive interventions and exacerbation of patient-level barriers. In addition, overdiagnosed cases of lung cancer may also increase, which are characterized as lung cancers that are detected by screening but that would otherwise have never been diagnosed and do not pose a threat to life. False-positive rate in the NLST reached 27% at baseline, 28% at the 1-year follow-up, and 16.6% at the 2-year follow-up,[79] which has since then decreased to nearly 5% secondary to implementation of Lung-reporting and data system (RADS).[80] Using various eligibility scenarios (different age groups, different smoking exposures) modeling, even the most advantageous eligibility strategy still led to 19.3% (19,300/100,000) of the population receiving false-positive results with 31.6% (910/2881) of the population with a positive screen undergoing biopsy or resection for benign lesions and 9.6% (190/1971) of cases detected by screening being overdiagnoses.[81] In a retrospective review of a radiography-based screening protocol in Italy, 14.2% (29/204) of benign lesions were diagnosed surgically.[82] Clearly, the implications of an optimally disseminated lung cancer screening program come with acceptable but significant drawbacks for health care systems and patient outcomes. A review of commonly misdiagnosed nodules may help identify a cohort of screened subjects that would most benefit from a blood-based adjunct in order to lessen the deleterious effects of a test with relatively low specificity (NLST specificity = 73.4%).

Although physical harms (unnecessary interventions) of lung cancer screening are routinely evaluated and reported, psychosocial stressors are not.[83] The work by Slatore and colleagues has showed that false positives in a lung screening program can lead to short-term increases in distress with an eventual return to baseline.[84] Given the elevated rate of false positives with the current screening standard, an adjunct to LDCT may help provide peace of mind to subjects with indeterminate- or low-risk findings that warrant continued radiographic observation.

Importantly, and depending on the role which a biomarker or liquid biopsy may serve, an optimal positive predictive value should be sought after in order to capture low-risk nodules that may be difficult to sample and could otherwise be early cancers. With improved sampling techniques, supplemented by biomarkers and/or liquid biopsy, ruling in indeterminate nodules may occur at a much higher rate, preventing the need for unnecessary invasive diagnostic tissue harvests.

FUTURE ROLES
Therapy Planning

Depending on the biomarker used to supplement LDCT lung cancer screening, data obtained from the liquid biopsy could provide insight on tumor-specific characteristics. These traits, in turn, can be used to personalize therapeutic strategies, including the potential for neoadjuvant therapy or eligibility in clinical trials. In addition, liquid biopsy, as an adjunct to LDCT, may provide real-time tumor information, ultimately guiding neoadjuvant treatment decisions.[85] Using such an approach that allows for genomic assessment can also predict resistance mutations to therapies.[86] Moreover, having access to a baseline measurement and serial tumor biomarker assessment may inform continuous dynamic risk profiling,[87] using pre- and post-therapy measurements, to ensure optimal personalized treatment plans for patients positively screened for lung cancer.

Disease Monitoring

Furthermore, liquid biopsy can also inform disease progression, recurrence, or response to neoadjuvant and adjuvant therapy.[88] Liquid biopsy (specifically ctDNA) has also been shown to be associated with oncologic outcomes such as progression-free survival.[89,90] Obtaining baseline measurements of these metrics via multimodal screening protocols may meaningfully augment our understanding of the dynamism of these biomarkers. With the advancement in current surgery-based multimodal therapy, there is an increase in minimal residual disease incidence. Liquid biopsy, in those cases, can be an incredibly valuable tool to survey disease recurrence.[91] Having access to a baseline measurement from the time of screening may be meaningful in the interpretation of subsequent biomarker assessments.

SUMMARY AND CONCLUSION

The current radiographic lung cancer screening protocol is an incredible endeavor capable of reducing cancer deaths. This benefit has been attributed to capturing and treating lung cancer during earlier stages of disease. However, there are some challenges met by the LDCT-based screening paradigm. First, uptake has been low; second, the rate of false positives remains very high. The potential of a liquid biopsy used to synergistically complement radiographic screening is tremendous. Not only can it encourage uptake in patients who may have borderline risk but it may also assuage the current rate of false positive by providing a personalized risk stratification.

CLINICS CARE POINTS

- Multiple modalities of blood-based assays are undergoing evaluation, standardization, and validation for diagnosis of lung cancer.
- As an adjunct to low-dose computed tomography, liquid biopsies and other biomarkers carry potential to increase accuracy and lower rate of false positives
- Blood-based assays for lung cancer can also provide insight on tumor characteristics and inform therapeutic strategy.

FUNDING

ND is supported by the Mason Family Philanthropic Fund. Rest of the authors have no relevant COI.

DISCLOSURE

The authors have nothing to disclose.

REFERENCES

1. Jemal A, Fedewa SA. Lung Cancer Screening With Low-Dose Computed Tomography in the United States-2010 to 2015. JAMA Oncol 2017;3(9):1278–81.
2. Vachani A, Carroll NM, Simoff MJ, et al. Stage Migration and Lung Cancer Incidence After Initiation of Low-Dose Computed Tomography Screening. J Thorac Oncol 2022;17(12):1355–64.
3. Raz DJ, Zell JA, Ou SH, et al. Natural history of stage I non-small cell lung cancer: implications for early detection. Chest 2007;132(1):193–9.
4. Khorana AA, Tullio K, Elson P, et al. Time to initial cancer treatment in the United States and association with survival over time: An observational study. PLoS One 2019;14(3):e0213209.
5. Ganti AK, Klein AB, Cotarla I, et al. Update of Incidence, Prevalence, Survival, and Initial Treatment in Patients With Non-Small Cell Lung Cancer in the US. JAMA Oncol 2021;7(12):1824–32.
6. Veronesi G, Bellomi M, Mulshine JL, et al. Lung cancer screening with low-dose computed tomography: A non-invasive diagnostic protocol for baseline lung nodules. Lung cancer (Amsterdam, Netherlands) 2008;61(3):340–9.
7. Aberle DR, Adams AM, Berg CD, et al. Reduced lung-cancer mortality with low-dose computed tomographic screening. N Engl J Med 2011;365(5):395–409.
8. de Koning HJ, van der Aalst CM, de Jong PA, et al. Reduced Lung-Cancer Mortality with Volume CT Screening in a Randomized Trial. N Engl J Med 2020;382(6):503–13.
9. Yang W, Qian F, Teng J, et al. Community-based lung cancer screening with low-dose CT in China: Results of the baseline screening. Lung Cancer 2018;117:20–6.
10. Moyer VA. U.S. Preventive Services Task Force. Screening for lung cancer: U.S. Preventive Services Task Force recommendation statement. Ann Intern Med 2014;160(5):330–8.
11. CMS. Decision Memo for Screening for Lung Cancer with Low-Dose Computed Tomography (LDCT) (CAG-00439N). 2015. Available at: https://www.cms.gov/medicare-coverage-database/view/ncacal-decision-memo.aspx?proposed=N&NCAId=274.
12. Force UPST. Screening for Lung Cancer: US Preventive Services Task Force Recommendation Statement. JAMA 2021;325(10):962–70.
13. Khouzam MS, Wood DE, Vigneswaran W, et al. Impact of Federal Lung Cancer Screening Policy on the Incidence of Early-Stage Lung Cancer. Ann Thorac Surg 2022;115(4):827–33.
14. Yong PC, Sigel K, Rehmani S, et al. Lung Cancer Screening Uptake in the United States. Chest 2020;157(1):236–8.
15. Association AL. State of Lung Cancer. 2023. Available at: https://www.lung.org/research/state-of-lung-cancer. Accessed January 24, 2023.
16. Triplette M, Thayer JH, Pipavath SN, et al. Poor Uptake of Lung Cancer Screening: Opportunities for Improvement. J Am Coll Radiol 2019;16(4):446–50.

17. Pleis JR, Coles R. Summary Health Statistics for US Adults: National Health Interview Survey: Department of Health and Human Services, Centers for Disease Control and …; 2009.

18. Li J, Chung S, Wei EK, et al. New recommendation and coverage of low-dose computed tomography for lung cancer screening: uptake has increased but is still low. BMC Health Serv Res 2018;18(1):525.

19. Atkins GT, Kim T, Munson J. Residence in Rural Areas of the United States and Lung Cancer Mortality. Disease Incidence, Treatment Disparities, and Stage-Specific Survival. Annals of the American Thoracic Society 2017;14(3):403–11.

20. Zgodic A, Zahnd WE, Advani S, et al. Low-dose CT lung cancer screening uptake: A rural–urban comparison. J Rural Health 2022;38(1):40–53.

21. Zahnd WE, James AS, Jenkins WD, et al. Rural-Urban Differences in Cancer Incidence and Trends in the United States. Cancer epidemiology 2018; 27(11):1265–74.

22. Johnson AM, Hines RB, Johnson JA 3rd, et al. Treatment and survival disparities in lung cancer: the effect of social environment and place of residence. Lung Cancer 2014;83(3):401–7.

23. Forrest LF, Adams J, Wareham H, et al. Socioeconomic inequalities in lung cancer treatment: systematic review and meta-analysis. PLoS Med 2013; 10(2):e1001376.

24. Dunlop KLA, Marshall HM, Stone E, et al. Motivation is not enough: A qualitative study of lung cancer screening uptake in Australia to inform future implementation. PLoS One 2022;17(9):e0275361–.

25. Quaife SL, Waller J, Dickson JL, et al. Psychological Targets for Lung Cancer Screening Uptake: A Prospective Longitudinal Cohort Study. J Thorac Oncol 2021;16(12):2016–28.

26. Rai A, Doria-Rose VP, Silvestri GA, et al. Evaluating Lung Cancer Screening Uptake, Outcomes, and Costs in the United States: Challenges With Existing Data and Recommendations for Improvement. J Natl Cancer Inst 2019;111(4):342–9.

27. Sestini S, Boeri M, Marchiano A, et al. Circulating microRNA signature as liquid-biopsy to monitor lung cancer in low-dose computed tomography screening. Oncotarget 2015;6(32):32868–77.

28. Freitas C, Sousa C, Machado F, et al. The Role of Liquid Biopsy in Early Diagnosis of Lung Cancer. Front Oncol 2021;11:634316.

29. Hofman V, Bonnetaud C, Ilie MI, et al. Preoperative circulating tumor cell detection using the isolation by size of epithelial tumor cell method for patients with lung cancer is a new prognostic biomarker. Clin Cancer Res 2011;17(4):827–35.

30. Bianchi F, Nicassio F, Marzi M, et al. A serum circulating miRNA diagnostic test to identify asymptomatic high-risk individuals with early stage lung cancer. EMBO Mol Med 2011;3(8):495–503.

31. Newman AM, Bratman SV, To J, et al. An ultrasensitive method for quantitating circulating tumor DNA with broad patient coverage. Nat Med 2014;20(5):548–54.

32. Tockman MS, Gupta PK, Myers JD, et al. Sensitive and specific monoclonal antibody recognition of human lung cancer antigen on preserved sputum cells: a new approach to early lung cancer detection. J Clin Oncol 1988;6(11):1685–93.

33. Dagogo-Jack IMD, Sequist L, Piotrowska ZMD. The Role of Liquid Biopsies in Lung Cancer Screening. Semin Roentgenol 2017;52(3):185–7.

34. Chabon JJ, Hamilton EG, Kurtz DM, et al. Integrating genomic features for non-invasive early lung cancer detection. Nature 2020;580(7802): 245–51.

35. Liu MC, Oxnard GR, Klein EA, et al. Sensitive and specific multi-cancer detection and localization using methylation signatures in cell-free DNA. Ann Oncol 2020;31(6):745–59.

36. Jamal-Hanjani M, Wilson GA, McGranahan N, et al. Tracking the Evolution of Non-Small-Cell Lung Cancer. N Engl J Med 2017;376(22): 2109–21.

37. Chaudhuri AA, Chabon JJ, Lovejoy AF, et al. Early Detection of Molecular Residual Disease in Localized Lung Cancer by Circulating Tumor DNA Profiling. Cancer Discov 2017;7(12):1394–403.

38. Siravegna G, Marsoni S, Siena S, et al. Integrating liquid biopsies into the management of cancer. Nat Rev Clin Oncol 2017;14(9):531–48.

39. Pastorino U, Boeri M, Sestini S, et al. Baseline computed tomography screening and blood microRNA predict lung cancer risk and define adequate intervals in the BioMILD trial. Ann Oncol 2022; 33(4):395–405.

40. Best MG, Wesseling P, Wurdinger T. Tumor-Educated Platelets as a Noninvasive Biomarker Source for Cancer Detection and Progression Monitoring. Cancer Res 2018;78(13):3407–12.

41. Antunes-Ferreira M, Koppers-Lalic D, Würdinger T. Circulating platelets as liquid biopsy sources for cancer detection. Mol Oncol 2021;15(6):1727–43.

42. Liu J, Ren L, Li S, et al. The biology, function, and applications of exosomes in cancer. Acta Pharm Sin B 2021;11(9):2783–97.

43. Cui S, Cheng Z, Qin W, et al. Exosomes as a liquid biopsy for lung cancer. Lung Cancer 2018;116: 46–54.

44. Sandúa A, Alegre E, González Á. Exosomes in Lung Cancer: Actors and Heralds of Tumor Development. Cancers 2021;13(17):4330.

45. Théry C, Witwer KW, Aikawa E, et al. Minimal information for studies of extracellular vesicles 2018 (MISEV2018): a position statement of the International Society for Extracellular Vesicles and update of the MISEV2014 guidelines. J Extracell Vesicles 2018;7(1):1535750.

46. Shin H, Oh S, Hong S, et al. Liquid biopsy of lung cancer by deep learning and spectroscopic analysis of circulating exosomes. J Clin Oncol 2020; 38(15_suppl):e15532–.

47. Tamminga M, Groen HJM, Hiltermann TJN. Circulating tumor cells as a liquid biopsy in small cell lung cancer, a future editorial. Transl Cancer Res 2017;6(S2):S353–6.

48. Hofman P. Liquid biopsy for lung cancer screening: Usefulness of circulating tumor cells and other circulating blood biomarkers. Cancer cytopathology 2021;129(5):341–6.

49. Singhal S, Rolfo C, Maksymiuk AW, et al. Liquid Biopsy in Lung Cancer Screening: The Contribution of Metabolomics. Results of A Pilot Study. Cancers 2019;11(8):1069.

50. Hanash SM, Ostrin EJ, Fahrmann JF. Blood based biomarkers beyond genomics for lung cancer screening. Transl Lung Cancer Res 2018;7(3): 327–35.

51. Ding Z, Wang N, Ji N, et al. Proteomics technologies for cancer liquid biopsies. Mol Cancer 2022;21(1): 53.

52. Dama E, Colangelo T, Fina E, et al. Biomarkers and Lung Cancer Early Detection: State of the Art. Cancers 2021;13(15):3919.

53. Murray A, Chapman CJ, Healey G, et al. Technical validation of an autoantibody test for lung cancer. Ann Oncol 2010;21(8):1687–93.

54. Boyle P, Chapman CJ, Holdenrieder S, et al. Clinical validation of an autoantibody test for lung cancer. Ann Oncol 2011;22(2):383–9.

55. Massion PP, Healey GF, Peek LJ, et al. Autoantibody Signature Enhances the Positive Predictive Power of Computed Tomography and Nodule-Based Risk Models for Detection of Lung Cancer. J Thorac Oncol 2017;12(3):578–84.

56. Jett JR, Peek LJ, Fredericks L, et al. Audit of the autoantibody test, EarlyCDT® -Lung, in 1600 patients: An evaluation of its performance in routine clinical practice. Lung cancer (Amsterdam, Netherlands) 2013;83(1):51–5.

57. Chapman CJ, Healey GF, Murray A, et al. EarlyCDT®-Lung test: improved clinical utility through additional autoantibody assays. Tumor Biol 2012; 33(5):1319–26.

58. Lam S, Boyle P, Healey GF, et al. EarlyCDT-Lung: an immunobiomarker test as an aid to early detection of lung cancer. Cancer Prev Res (Philadelphia, Pa) 2011;4(7):1126–34.

59. Li X-j, Hayward C, Fong P-Y, et al. A blood-based proteomic classifier for the molecular characterization of pulmonary nodules. Sci Transl Med 2013; 5(207). 207ra142-207ra142.

60. Ostrin EJ, Sidransky D, Spira A, et al. Biomarkers for Lung Cancer Screening and Detection. Cancer Epidemiol Biomarkers Prev 2020;29(12):2411–5.

61. Raval AA, Benn BS, Benzaquen S, et al. Reclassification of risk of malignancy with Percepta Genomic Sequencing Classifier following nondiagnostic bronchoscopy. Respir Med 2022;204:106990.

62. Lee HJ, Mazzone P, Feller-Kopman D, et al. Impact of the Percepta Genomic Classifier on Clinical Management Decisions in a Multicenter Prospective Study. Chest 2021;159(1):401–12.

63. Salvi S, Gurioli G, De Giorgi U, et al. Cell-free DNA as a diagnostic marker for cancer: current insights. OncoTargets Ther 2016;9:6549–59.

64. Corcoran RB, Chabner BA. Application of Cell-free DNA Analysis to Cancer Treatment. N Engl J Med 2018;379(18):1754–65.

65. Klein EA, Richards D, Cohn A, et al. Clinical validation of a targeted methylation-based multi-cancer early detection test using an independent validation set. Ann Oncol 2021;32(9):1167–77.

66. Qi T, Pan M, Shi H, et al. Cell-Free DNA Fragmentomics: The Novel Promising Biomarker. Int J Mol Sci 2023;24(2):1503.

67. Liu Y. At the dawn: cell-free DNA fragmentomics and gene regulation. Br J Cancer 2022;126(3):379–90.

68. Cristiano S, Leal A, Phallen J, et al. Genome-wide cell-free DNA fragmentation in patients with cancer. Nature 2019;570(7761):385–9.

69. Tammemägi MC, Katki HA, Hocking WG, et al. Selection Criteria for Lung-Cancer Screening. N Engl J Med 2013;368(8):728–36.

70. Fahrmann JF, Marsh T, Irajizad E, et al. Blood-Based Biomarker Panel for Personalized Lung Cancer Risk Assessment. J Clin Oncol 2022;40(8):876–83.

71. Ostrin EJ, Bantis LE, Wilson DO, et al. Contribution of a Blood-Based Protein Biomarker Panel to the Classification of Indeterminate Pulmonary Nodules. J Thorac Oncol 2021;16(2):228–36.

72. Aldrich MC, Mercaldo SF, Sandler KL, et al. Evaluation of USPSTF Lung Cancer Screening Guidelines Among African American Adult Smokers. JAMA Oncol 2019;5(9):1318–24.

73. Fedewa SA, Kazerooni EA, Studts JL, et al. State Variation in Low-Dose Computed Tomography Scanning for Lung Cancer Screening in the United States. J Natl Cancer Inst 2021;113(8):1044–52.

74. Haddad DN, Sandler KL, Henderson LM, et al. Disparities in Lung Cancer Screening: A Review. Ann Am Thorac Soc 2020;17(4):399–405.

75. Pinsky PF, Lau YK, Doubeni CA. Potential Disparities by Sex and Race or Ethnicity in Lung Cancer Screening Eligibility Rates. Chest 2021;160(1): 341–50.

76. Sahar L, Douangchai Wills VL, Liu KK, et al. Geographic access to lung cancer screening among eligible adults living in rural and urban environments in the United States. Cancer 2022;128(8):1584–94.

77. Zarei Jalalabadi N, Rahimi B, Foroumandi M, et al. Willingness to participate in a lung cancer screening

program: Patients' attitudes towards United States Preventive Services Taskforce (USPSTF) recommendations. Eur J Intern Med 2022;98:128–9.

78. Meza R, Jeon J, Toumazis I, et al. Evaluation of the Benefits and Harms of Lung Cancer Screening With Low-Dose Computed Tomography: Modeling Study for the US Preventive Services Task Force. JAMA, J Am Med Assoc 2021;325(10):988–97.

79. Hirsch FRP, Scagliotti GVP, Mulshine JLP, et al. Lung cancer: current therapies and new targeted treatments. Lancet (British edition) 2016;389(10066): 299–311.

80. Pinsky PF, Gierada DS, Black W, et al. Performance of Lung-RADS in the National Lung Screening Trial: a retrospective assessment. Ann Intern Med 2015; 162(7):485–91.

81. de Koning H, Meza R, Plevritis SK, et al. Benefits and Harms of Computed Tomography Lung Cancer Screening Strategies: A Comparative Modeling Study for the US Preventive Services Task Force. Ann Intern Med 2014;160(5):311–+.

82. Veronesi G, Maisonneuve P, Spaggiari L, et al. Diagnostic Performance of Low-Dose Computed Tomography Screening for Lung Cancer over Five Years. J Thorac Oncol 2014;9(7):935–9.

83. Menezes R, Roberts H. Lung Cancer Screening Using Low-Dose Computed Tomography—Keeping Participants Out of Harm's Way. J Thorac Oncol 2014;9(7):912–3.

84. Slatore CG, Sullivan DR, Pappas M, et al. Patient-centered outcomes among lung cancer screening recipients with computed tomography: a systematic review. J Thorac Oncol 2014;9(7):927–34.

85. Zhou E, Li Y, Wu F, et al. Circulating extracellular vesicles are effective biomarkers for predicting response to cancer therapy. EBioMedicine 2021; 67:103365.

86. Liam CK, Mallawathantri S, Fong KM. Is tissue still the issue in detecting molecular alterations in lung cancer? Respirology 2020;25(9):933–43.

87. Kurtz DM, Esfahani MS, Scherer F, et al. Dynamic Risk Profiling Using Serial Tumor Biomarkers for Personalized Outcome Prediction. Cell 2019; 178(3):699–713.e19.

88. Yi C, He Y, Xia H, et al. Review and perspective on adjuvant and neoadjuvant immunotherapies in NSCLC. OncoTargets Ther 2019;12:7329–36.

89. Romero A, Nadal E, Serna R, et al. OA20.02 Pre-Treatment Levels of ctDNA for Long-Term Survival Prediction in Stage IIIA NSCLC Treated With Neoadjuvant Chemo-Immunotherapy. J Thorac Oncol 2021;16(10):S883–4.

90. Forde PM, Spicer J, Lu S, et al. Neoadjuvant Nivolumab plus Chemotherapy in Resectable Lung Cancer. N Engl J Med 2022;386(21):1973–85.

91. Pantel K, Alix-Panabières C. Liquid biopsy and minimal residual disease - latest advances and implications for cure. Nat Rev Clin Oncol 2019;16(7):409–24.

Clinical Adjuncts to Lung Cancer Screening
A Narrative Review

Cynthia J. Susai, MD[a], Jeffrey B. Velotta, MD[b], Lori C. Sakoda, PhD, MPH[c],*

KEYWORDS

- Lung cancer screening • Risk prediction • Shared-decision-making • Biomarkers

KEY POINTS

- The benefit-to-harm ratio associated with lung cancer screening (LCS) varies considerably among screening eligible individuals.
- Clinical adjuncts can be used to tailor and guide decision-making at key steps to improving LCS effectiveness and efficiency.
- Although many proposed adjuncts to LCS seem beneficial, further evidence is needed regarding their clinical utility and implementation to support their use in practice.

BACKGROUND

With the 2021 update of the US Preventive Services Task Force (USPSTF) lung cancer screening (LCS) guidelines, the population eligible for LCS with low-dose computed tomography (LDCT) expanded by 87%, enabling more women and racial/ethnic minority individuals to benefit from screening.[1,2] The guidelines recommend screening based on age (50–80 years) and smoking history (≥20 pack-years and smoked within the past 15 years).[2] However, among the screening eligible population, the individual risk of lung cancer is highly heterogeneous, and the mortality benefit associated with screening varies based on lung cancer risk.[3] Without considering other factors, including comorbidities and life expectancy, this approach inherently includes individuals who are unlikely to benefit from screening and excludes individuals who are more likely to benefit from screening.[4] An alternate approach is to tailor screening based on a more personalized risk assessment to improve the balance of benefits to harms.

In this context, clinical adjuncts, or additional information and tools to guide clinical decision-making, may optimize LCS effectiveness and efficiency. Proposed adjunctive approaches integrate clinical history, risk prediction models, shared decision-making (SDM) tools, and biomarker tests, with varying applicability to current practice. These clinical adjuncts can guide key steps in LCS, including selecting screening candidates, supporting SDM, evaluating screening-detected nodules for cancer, and determining screening intervals (**Fig. 1**). Herein, we review the most promising clinical adjuncts and highlight where in the screening process they may be most useful.

DISCUSSION
Clinical History

Perhaps most notably missing from LCS guidelines is consideration of family history and medical history. Family history of lung cancer is known to increase the risk for the disease, independent of smoking history.[5] However, family history in the clinical context tends to include only first-degree relatives and often suffers from accurate recall, leading to a less precise calculation of risk. In a study estimating lung cancer risk based on complete family history from linked statewide cancer registry data and genealogy records, individuals

a UCSF East Bay General Surgery, 1411 East 31st Street QIC 22134, Oakland, CA 94612, USA; b Department of Thoracic Surgery, Kaiser Permanente Northern California, 3600 Broadway, Oakland, CA 94611, USA; c Division of Research, Kaiser Permanente Northern California, 2000 Broadway, Oakland, CA 94612, USA
* Corresponding author.
E-mail address: lori.sakoda@kp.org

Thorac Surg Clin 33 (2023) 421–432
https://doi.org/10.1016/j.thorsurg.2023.03.002
1547-4127/23/© 2023 Elsevier Inc. All rights reserved.

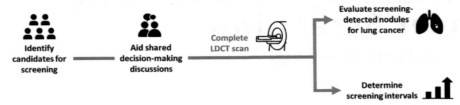

Fig. 1. Potential use of clinical adjuncts at key steps in LCS.

at two to five-fold higher risk for lung cancer were identified.[6] Therefore, with additional family history data, better risk calculations could be performed to inform decisions about LCS.

Beyond recommending against screening individuals with a health condition that substantially limits life expectancy or the ability to undergo curative lung surgery, the USPSTF provides little guidance on screening individuals with comorbidities.[2] Chronic obstructive pulmonary disease (COPD) is a major risk factor for lung cancer, noted in 60% to 85% of cases.[7] Screening eligible individuals at greatest risk for lung cancer have the highest prevalence of COPD and a higher risk of dying from other causes, due to a high prevalence of cardiovascular and other chronic diseases.[7,8] Accordingly, those with COPD at utmost lung cancer risk may not actually benefit from LCS. In a National Lung Screening Trial (NLST) sub-analysis, the benefit of annual LCS was greatest in those with normal lung function or mild-to-moderate COPD, not in those with severe or very severe COPD.[8] A limitation of using the degree of COPD severity to recommend LCS is that individuals would need spirometry before LDCT. However, routine in-office spirometry may help to identify those with airflow limitation who are more likely to benefit from LCS.

Other lung-specific comorbidities, including emphysema and interstitial lung disease, also confer lung cancer risk.[9,10] Even non-primary lung disease, such as peripheral arterial disease, has been associated with increased lung cancer risk, likely because smoking history is a shared risk factor. The extent to which existing comorbidities may be incorporated into estimating the benefits and harms of LCS is relatively unknown, warranting further investigation.[11]

Risk Prediction Models

Proposed risk prediction models estimate the probability of developing or dying from lung cancer or the probability of pulmonary nodule malignancy, based on age, smoking history, and other clinical and non-clinical factors. These models can be applied at each step in **Fig. 1** to optimize screening efficiency and outcomes.

To be clinically useful, a risk prediction model should be accurate, reliable, and generalizable to its target population. A model may underperform when applied to populations independent from which it was developed, because of shortcomings in its development or variation in population composition or predictor variable measurement.[12] External validation of a model's predictive performance is therefore necessary before it is used clinically. Predictive performance is commonly evaluated by discrimination and calibration. Discrimination, often quantified by the area under the curve (AUC), indicates the ability of a model to accurately classify individuals with or without the event of interest, while calibration indicates the closeness between the probabilities of model-predicted or expected (E) versus observed (O) events. Even if a model discriminates well (high AUC), it is impractical if it is insufficiently calibrated (E/O ratio far below or above 1.0). Accordingly, we focus on models that have been externally validated in independent populations.

Predicting lung cancer risk before screening. Applying risk prediction models to select high-risk individuals for LCS could improve the balance of benefits to harms by screening fewer individuals, discovering fewer false-positive results, and detecting more early-stage lung cancers. Over 30 distinct models have been proposed to predict individual risk of developing or dying from lung cancer within a specified time frame.[13] The majority predict risk based on age, smoking history, and other conventional risk factors, including sex, family history of lung cancer, and COPD or emphysema. Some incorporate additional factors requiring clinical assessment (eg, lung function measures) or biospecimen collection and analysis (eg, molecular and genetic markers).

To date, less than half of these models have been externally validated, primarily those incorporating only conventional risk factors, of which five have performed relatively well in United States, European, and Australian cohorts (**Table 1**).[14–21] Four of these models are derived from US trial populations, specifically the Bach model in the Carotene and Retinol Efficacy Trial (CARET) population of high-risk smokers and the PLCO$_{M2012}$

Table 1
Externally validated top-performing models predicting risk of lung cancer incidence or mortality

Model [Reference]	Location Data Source(s)	Outcome	Target Population	Predictors	Predictive Performance
Bach et al,[22] 2003	United States • CARET: 18,172 high-risk smokers	Lung cancer incidence in 1 y	Ever-smoking adults	Age; sex; smoking intensity, duration, and quit-years; asbestos exposure	AUC: 0.72 Calibration assessed graphically
PLCO$_{M2012}$[23]	United States Development: • 36,286 PLCO control arm smokers aged 55–74 Validation: • 37,332 PLCO intervention arm smokers aged 55–74 • 51,033 NLST participants	Lung cancer incidence in 6 y	Ever-smoking adults	Age; education; race/ethnicity; BMI; smoking status, intensity, duration, and quit-years; COPD; history of cancer; family history of lung cancer	AUC: 0.797 (PLCO), 0.701 (NLST) Calibration: 90th percentile absolute error = 0.042
LCRAT[24]	United States Development: • 39,180 PLCO control arm smokers aged 55–74 Validation: • 39,822 PLCO intervention arm smokers aged 55–74 • 26,554 NLST control arm participants	Lung cancer incidence in 5 y	Ever-smoking adults	Age; sex; education; race/ethnicity; BMI; smoking intensity, duration, pack-years, and quit-years; emphysema; family history of lung cancer	AUC: 0.80 (PLCO), 0.70 (NLST) E/O: 0.94 (PLCO), 1.06 (NLST)

(continued on next page)

Table 1
(continued)

Model [Reference]	Location Data Source(s)	Outcome	Target Population	Predictors	Predictive Performance
LCDRAT[24]	United States Development: • 39,180 PLCO control arm smokers aged 55–74 Validation: • 39,822 PLCO intervention arm smokers aged 55–74 • 26,554 NLST control arm participants • 29,091 NHIS smokers aged 50–80	Lung cancer mortality in 5 y	Ever-smoking adults	Age; sex; education; race/ethnicity; BMI; smoking intensity, duration, pack-years, and quit-years; emphysema; family history of lung cancer	AUC: 0.81 (PLCO), 0.73 (NLST), 0.78 (NHIS) E/O: 1.08 (PLCO), 1.31 (NLST), 0.94 (NHIS)
LLP[25]	United Kingdom Age- and sex-matched case-control study: 579 lung cancer cases, 1157 controls	Lung cancer incidence in 5 y	General population	Smoking duration; asbestos exposure; history of pneumonia; history of cancer; family history of lung cancer	AUC: 0.70 Calibration not assessed
LLP$_{v2}$[26]	United Kingdom Age- and sex-matched case-control study: 579 lung cancer cases, 1157 controls	Lung cancer incidence in 5 y	Ever-smoking adults	Smoking duration; asbestos exposure; history of pneumonia; history of emphysema; history of bronchitis; history of tuberculosis; history of COPD; history of cancer; family history of lung cancer	Not reported

model, Lung Cancer Risk Assessment Tool (LCRAT), and Lung Cancer Death Risk Assessment Tool (LCDRAT) in the Prostate, Lung, Colorectal, and Ovarian (PLCO) Screening Trial and NLST populations of ever-smokers. The Bach model is the simplest, incorporating age, sex, asbestos exposure, and smoking intensity, duration and quit-years to estimate annual lung cancer incidence.[22] The $PLCO_{M2012}$ model incorporates age, race/ethnicity, education, body mass index (BMI), COPD, history of cancer, family history of lung cancer, and smoking status, intensity, duration, and quit-years to predict a 6-year lung cancer incidence.[23] LCRAT and LCDRAT include the same set of predictors (age, sex, education, race/ethnicity, BMI, emphysema, family history of lung cancer, and smoking intensity, duration, and quit-years) to estimate a 5-year lung cancer incidence or mortality, respectively.[24] In contrast, the Liverpool Lung Project (LLP) model was derived from a matched case-control study population in the United Kingdom, including never-smoking individuals, to predict a 5-year lung cancer incidence based on smoking duration, asbestos exposure, history of pneumonia, history of cancer, and family history of lung cancer.[25] It has been since updated (LLP_{v2}) to incorporate a history of other respiratory diseases and limited to ever-smoking individuals.[26]

Using well-validated risk prediction models to select ever-smoking individuals for LCS is more effective in preventing lung cancer deaths compared with USPSTF screening criteria.[23,24] In LCS trials outside the United States, the $PLCO_{M2012}$ and LLP_{v2} models have and are being applied to optimize the selection of high-risk individuals.[26–28] Applying risk prediction models may additionally reduce lung cancer disparities. In retrospective analyses, the $PLCO_{M2012}$ model had a higher sensitivity for detecting lung cancer, especially among African Americans and women, over the USPSTF LCS criteria.[29,30]

From a cost-effectiveness perspective, however, the value of risk-based screening seems modest.[31] Despite efficiency in averting more lung cancer deaths per person screened, risk-based screening preferentially selects those at the highest risk, who are generally older, smoke heavier, and have more comorbidities. Those at the highest risk, in turn, are costlier to screen and may benefit less due to shorter life expectancy. To address these concerns, novel strategies that consider estimated gains in life expectancy and individual preferences have been proposed.[32–34] Although screening high-risk individuals with long life expectancy is preferable, the minimum gain in life expectancy by which to recommend screening remains less clear.

Predicting nodule malignancy risk. Using risk prediction models that accurately distinguish malignant from benign pulmonary nodules may facilitate earlier lung cancer diagnosis and treatment and reduce harms and costs from unnecessary follow-up. Currently, the Lung CT Screening Reporting and Data System (Lung-RADS) is used in the United States to standardize the interpretation and management of LDCT screening results.[35] Results are classified visually into assessment categories that define whether a screening examination is negative (category 1 or 2) or positive (category 3 or 4 A/B/X).

Table 2 presents the most commonly validated models for predicting pulmonary nodule malignancy. These models are derived from patient populations across diverse settings and malignancy prevalence and incorporate different combinations of patient and imaging characteristics. The Mayo Clinic and veterans affairs (VA) models were originally constructed to estimate the pretest probability of malignancy for solitary pulmonary nodules (SPN) detected incidentally by chest radiography.[36,37] The Peking University People's Hospital (PKUPH) model was later developed and shown to predict nodule malignancy risk more accurately than the Mayo Clinic and VA models among Chinese patients.[38] In comparison, the Brock (PanCan) model is the only one developed using trial data to estimate the malignancy risk of screen-detected pulmonary nodules among ever-smoking patients.[39]

These models have generally performed less well than originally reported across independent external validation studies. In most studies comparing the Brock model to others in non-screening populations, the discriminatory accuracy of the Brock model has been greater or equivalent to that of the Mayo Clinic model, yet greater than the VA and PKUPH models.[40–44] In the largest and most recent evaluation, however, the Mayo Clinic model exhibited greater accuracy than the Brock model in discriminating malignancy risk of large (>8 mm) nodules.[45] Across studies that also assessed calibration, both models underestimated or overestimated the actual probability of malignancy.[42,43,45] In the only study to compare these four models in a screening population, the Brock model performed best, exhibiting excellent discrimination and acceptable calibration.[46] Yet, data are inconsistent on whether the Brock model outperforms Lung-RADS in discriminating malignancy risk for screening-detected nodules.[47,48] Overall, existing prediction models seem to be of limited utility in optimizing nodule management at present.

Predicting lung cancer risk to optimize screening intervals. Several lung cancer risk prediction models

Table 2
Externally validated models predicting risk of pulmonary nodule malignancy

Model [Reference]	Location Data Source(s)	Malignancy Prevalence	Predictors	Predictive Performance
Mayo[36]	United States 629 Mayo Clinic patients with indeterminate 4–30 mm SPN found by chest radiography	23%	Age; smoking status; history of extrathoracic cancer; nodule diameter, spiculation, location	AUC: 0.80 Hosmer-Lemeshow goodness of fit, $P = .62$
VA[37]	United States 375 VA patients with 7–30 mm SPN found by chest radiography	54%	Age; smoking status and quit-years; nodule diameter	AUC: 0.78 Hosmer-Lemeshow goodness of fit, $P = .61$
PKUPH[38]	China Development: 371 patients with pathologically diagnosed SPN from 2000 to 2009 Validation: 62 patients with pathologically diagnosed SPN from 2009 to 2010	53%	Age; family history of cancer; nodule diameter, spiculation, border, calcification	AUC: 0.89 Calibration not assessed
Brock (PanCan)[39]	Canada Development: 1871 high-risk smokers with nodules from PanCan Study Validation: 1090 high-risk smokers with nodules from BCCA chemoprevention trials	PanCan: 5.5% BCCA: 3.7%	Age; sex; family history of lung cancer; emphysema; nodule diameter, spiculation, location, type, count	AUC >0.90 Calibration: 90th percentile absolute error = 0.003

have been extended by incorporating LDCT results to determine optimal screening intervals. Using the Continuous Observation of Smoking Subject (COSMOS) trial data, Maisonneuve and colleagues recalibrated and extended the Bach model to include lung nodule characteristics and emphysema identified at the baseline screening examination as predictors.[49] When externally validated in ever-smoking individuals receiving annual LCS for 10 years, this model showed an accurate prediction of lung cancer for the first two screening rounds, but overprediction thereafter.[50] Using data from independent sets of NLST participants, Tammemägi and colleagues developed and validated the PLCO$_{M2012}$ results model, which added Lung-RADS results to the PLCO$_{M2012}$ model.[51] Also with the NLST data, Robbins and colleagues developed the LCRAT + CT model to continuously predict short-term lung cancer risk following a negative or positive LDCT examination, as a function of pre-screening risk factors (LCRAT) and LDCT features[52]; this model has not yet been externally validated. Applying risk prediction models to personalize follow-up based on LDCT results could increase LCS efficiency and cost-effectiveness, but this remains to be proven.

Further Considerations. Although evidence suggests integrating risk prediction models into LCS can avert more lung cancer deaths and reduce unnecessary follow-up procedures and costs, additional considerations are important to recognize before implementation (**Box 1**).

Shared Decision-Making Tools

Individual preferences must be respected, given the US Centers for Medicare and Medicaid Services coverage requirement for SDM before LDCT screening.[34] Conveying the risks, benefits, and uncertainties of LCS to individuals requires a complex SDM conversation. SDM tools vary in the method of delivery, from classroom exercises, handouts, surveys, or web-based tools.[58,59] Overall, a systematic review of 15 such tools demonstrated increased patient knowledge and decreased decisional conflict.[58]

Web-based SDM tools are increasingly common. The important factors in determining if such tools will improve decision-making include ease of use, integration into the electronic medical record (EMR), and comprehensibility. LCSDesTool, one web-based tool in the VA system, provided usability but faltered in comprehensibility secondary to medical jargon.[60] Another tool used in the VA population, DecisionPrecision, suffered from poor EMR integration, worsening time constraints for primary care providers.[61] Some tools have

integrated lung cancer risk calculators, for example, shouldiscreen.com that calculates risk with the PLCO$_{M2012}$ model, although the individual risk calculated and depicted by these tools varies considerably.[62] In a prospective randomized control trial, shouldiscreen.com was compared with Options Grids, a one-page summary table to compare the options, with frequently asked questions for each option. Though evidence suggested both tools facilitated a high-quality SDM process, Options Grids was associated with decreased decision regret and increased patient knowledge.[63] As these tools are integrated into clinical practice, their constant improvement and evaluation will serve to improve the quality of SDM conversations going forward.

Biomarkers

Significant efforts also focus on discovering and validating biomarkers as a complement to LDCT in identifying individuals who are more likely to benefit from LCS and discriminating benign from malignant nodules seen at imaging. Although numerous different biomarkers have been evaluated, their clinical utility remains insufficiently investigated. We highlight those biomarker tests used in clinical practice currently, as many others are at various stages of research and development.[64,65]

Post-Screening Biomarkers

More biomarker tests have been validated and have become commercially available in the diagnostic setting, namely in determining the malignancy risk of indeterminate pulmonary nodules. One example is EarlyCDT-Lung (Onc-Immune). This blood test measures autoantibodies against p53, cancer-associated gene protein (CAGE), New York esophageal squamous cell carcinoma 1 (NY-ESO-1), SRY-box transcription factor 2 (SOX2), GBU4-5, ELAV-like protein 4 (HuD), and melanoma-associated antigen A4 (MAGE-A4) to assess pulmonary nodule malignancy risk, although it has been evaluated for use in the early detection of lung cancer.[66] In a double-blinded randomized trial comparing the use of EarlyCDT-Lung followed by LDCT to usual care, EarlyCDT-Lung detected lung cancers at an earlier stage, but did not increase the frequency of lung cancer detection over 2 years.[67] Another protein-based assay "PAULA's" test (Protein Assays Utilizing Lung cancer Analytes), which measures carcinoembryonic antigen (CEA), cancer antigen 125 (CA-125), cytokeratin 19 fragment antigen 21-1 (CYFRA 21-1), and New York esophageal squamous cell carcinoma 1 (NY-ESO-1) to detect lung cancer in high-risk individuals, was able to

---

Box 1
Further considerations for clinical implementation of risk prediction models

1. *Determining benefits and harms of using risk prediction models.* Simulation studies indicate that risk prediction models may be more effective in determining screening eligibility than existing age and smoking history criteria; yet, empirical data are limited on whether a risk-tailored approach improves lung cancer detection and outcomes.[2] Prospective studies enrolling individuals using risk prediction models will offer insight into the effectiveness and feasibility of this approach. The International Lung Screening Trial (ILST) is evaluating the accuracy of the PLCO$_{M2012}$ model versus USPSTF eligibility criteria in detecting lung cancers and the efficiency of the PanCan model versus Lung-RADS in managing screen-detected nodules.[28] Based on interim and economic analyses of ILST data, the PLCO$_{M2012}$ model seems to be more efficient and cost-effective than the 2013 USPSTF criteria in selecting screening candidates.[53,54] The Yorkshire Lung Screening Trial has similar plans to compare outcomes between individuals selected using the PLCO$_{M2012}$ model, LLPv2 model, and 2013 USPSTF criteria.[27]

2. *Demonstrating clinical feasibility and acceptability.* The USPSTF has called for studies to identify implementation barriers associated with risk-tailored screening, given uncertainty about how using risk prediction models could hinder LCS implementation in primary care.[2] Model-based risk assessment is more complex, requiring information beyond age and smoking history. Although yet unproven, automating risk model calculations within electronic health records may feasibly support personalized LCS programs.[55] Models requiring any information from clinical or biomarker assessment, especially if not readily available or measurable, may thus be impractical, even if they demonstrate better predictive performance. Also, as some models include race and socioeconomic status, their acceptability in calculating lung cancer risk and life expectancy should be examined.[55]

3. *Identifying optimal thresholds.* No consensus exists on the cost-effective threshold for personalized selection of ever-smoking individuals in LCS. The proposed PLCO$_{M2012}$ risk threshold of 1.51% was based on where lung cancer mortality was consistently lower among NLST intervention versus control participants and not on cost-effectiveness.[56] As risk models seem to yield different absolute risk estimates for the same individual,[17] optimal risk thresholds must be specified for each model.

4. *Broadening scope to never-smoking individuals.* In western countries, the potential application of personalized LCS has focused on ever-smoking individuals. To broaden LCS to the general population, more extensive research would be needed to determine the accuracy of risk assessment and cost-effectiveness of screening never-smoking individuals.[57]

---

distinguish cases from controls with 77% sensitivity, 80% specificity, and 0.85 AUC in the independent validation phase.[68] Although serum protein-based assays show great promise, further study is needed to determine their clinical validity.

Exhaled breath condensate (EBC) is another source to sample the airway specifically. EBC contains cells, DNA fragments, and volatile organic compounds. These compounds can be analyzed by mass spectrometry, nano-sensors, and colorimetric sensors. EBC analysis has been shown to be helpful in discerning between benign and malignant pulmonary nodules and predicting response to therapy, but has not demonstrated utility in determining whom to screen.[69,70]

Bronchoscopy samples are another avenue to detect genetic alterations caused by cigarette smoking damage to the respiratory tract epithelium. A 2007 study first demonstrated an 80-gene expression set measured from histologically normal bronchial airway brushings could differentiate smokers with and without lung cancer at 90% sensitivity and 84% specificity.[71] In two large prospective multicenter trials of patients undergoing bronchoscopy for concern of lung cancer, this airway gene expression classifier showed similar sensitivity (88%–89%), which increased when combined with bronchoscopy (96%–98%), but lower specificity (47% in both).[72] The test proved useful when bronchoscopy was nondiagnostic, as the classifier had a 91% negative predictive value in patients with an intermediate pre-bronchoscopy probability of cancer and a negative bronchoscopy. Compared with other tests, the Percepta Genomic Sequencing Classifier introduced clinically in 2015 and updated in 2019, primarily assists with lung cancer risk stratification when bronchoscopy is inconclusive.[73,74] Its clinical importance will be elucidated even more with ongoing use, including in the LCS context.

Pre-screening Biomarkers

There are also biomarker tests for determining lung cancer risk, but none are currently approved for clinical use. An avenue for increasing early lung cancer detection is analyzing the circulating genetic material. Among the most promising is the use of cell-free DNA (cfDNA) to non-invasively detect lung cancer. One novel approach called the DNA evaluation of fragments for early interception (DELFI) applies machine-learning algorithms to identify genome-wide cfDNA fragmentation profiles associated with cancer.[75] A large, multisite prospective validation study (Cancer Screening Assay using DELPHI [CASCADE]-LUNG, NCT05306288) is currently evaluating its performance in detecting lung cancer among screening eligible individuals.

Other biomarkers include microRNAs (miRNAs), a family of molecules that help regulate gene expression. Two different tests, the miRNA signature classifier and the Mi-R test, were shown to decrease LDCT-false-positive rates by five-fold and four-fold (while maintaining specificity and sensitivity above 75%), respectively, in two large retrospective studies from Italy.[76,77] As malignant cells are likewise found in sputum, a sputum-based test (LuCED) has been developed that detects abnormal bronchial epithelial cells using a novel imaging technology followed by a cytopathologist review.[78] Also as whole genome sequencing costs have declined, more attention has shifted toward using genetics to risk stratify individuals using polygenic risk scores (PRS). In a recent analysis, trajectories of five-years and cumulative absolute risk for lung cancer varied between individuals at different PRS deciles, suggesting that genetic background could be used to more efficiently tailor LCS.[79]

SUMMARY

Clinical adjuncts represent a promising opportunity to improve LCS effectiveness and efficiency by tailoring and guiding clinical decision-making. Adjunctive use of clinical history, risk prediction models, and SDM tools has been considered most in optimizing the selection of screening candidates and SDM. Currently, biomarker tests are only available clinically for pulmonary nodule evaluation. Although many proposed adjuncts to LCS seem beneficial, further evidence is needed regarding their clinical utility and implementation to support their use in practice.

CLINICS CARE POINTS

- Lung cancer risk is heterogeneous among screening eligible individuals.
- The mortality benefit associated with LCS is greater among individuals at higher lung cancer risk. However, those at the highest risk may not benefit from LCS, given lower life expectancy and higher mortality from other causes.

- Decisions to recommend LCS should assess lung cancer risk, life expectancy, and personal preferences. Well-validated risk prediction and SDM tools can support this process, although best practices have yet to be established.
- Although biomarkers may be integrated with LDCT to improve the selection of individuals who are likely to benefit from LCS and discrimination of indeterminate pulmonary nodules, biomarker tests are only presently available to aid with pulmonary nodule evaluation.
- USPSTF guidelines recommend LCS based on age and smoking history. Individuals identified using clinical adjuncts who do not meet USPSTF criteria may incur issues with LCS reimbursement.

DISCLOSURE

L.C. Sakoda has received funding for research on lung cancer from AstraZeneca, United States, paid directly to her institution.

REFERENCES

1. Meza R, Jeon J, Toumazis I, et al. Evaluation of the benefits and harms of lung cancer screening with low-dose computed tomography: modeling study for the US Preventive Services Task Force. JAMA 2021;325(10):988–97.
2. Krist AH, Davidson KW, Mangione CM, et al. Screening for lung cancer: US Preventive Services Task Force recommendation statement. JAMA 2021;325(10):962–70.
3. Jonas DE, Reuland DS, Reddy SM, et al. Screening for lung cancer with low-dose computed tomography: updated evidence report and systematic review for the US Preventive Services Task Force. JAMA 2021;325(10):971–87.
4. Katki HA, Cheung LC, Landy R. Basing eligibility for lung cancer screening on individualized risk calculators should save more lives, but life expectancy matters. J Natl Cancer Inst 2020;112(5):429–30.
5. Coté ML, Liu M, Bonassi S, et al. Increased risk of lung cancer in individuals with a family history of the disease: a pooled analysis from the International Lung Cancer Consortium. Eur J Cancer 2012; 48(13):1957–68.
6. Cannon-Albright LA, Carr SR, Akerley W. Population-based relative risks for lung cancer based on complete family history of lung cancer. J Thorac Oncol 2019;14(7):1184–91.
7. Young RP, Hopkins RJ. Chronic obstructive pulmonary disease (COPD) and lung cancer screening. Transl Lung Cancer Res 2018;7(3):347–60.

8. Hopkins RJ, Duan F, Chiles C, et al. Reduced expiratory flow rate among heavy smokers increases lung cancer risk. results from the National Lung Screening Trial-American College of Radiology Imaging Network cohort. Ann Am Thorac Soc 2017; 14(3):392–402.

9. González J, Henschke CI, Yankelevitz DF, et al. Emphysema phenotypes and lung cancer risk. PLoS One 2019;14(7):e0219187.

10. Whittaker Brown SA, Padilla M, Mhango G, et al. Interstitial lung abnormalities and lung cancer risk in the national lung screening trial. Chest 2019; 156(6):1195–203.

11. Rivera MP, Tanner NT, Silvestri GA, et al. Incorporating coexisting chronic illness into decisions about patient selection for lung cancer screening. An official American thoracic society research statement. Am J Respir Crit Care Med 2018;198(2):e3–13.

12. Altman DG, Vergouwe Y, Royston P, Moons KG. Prognosis and prognostic research: validating a prognostic model. BMJ 2009;338:b605.

13. Toumazis I, Bastani M, Han SS, Plevritis SK. Risk-based lung cancer screening: A systematic review. Lung Cancer 2020;147:154–86.

14. D'Amelio AM Jr, Cassidy A, Asomaning K, et al. Comparison of discriminatory power and accuracy of three lung cancer risk models. Br J Cancer 2010;103(3):423–9.

15. Raji OY, Duffy SW, Agbaje OF, et al. Predictive accuracy of the Liverpool Lung Project risk model for stratifying patients for computed tomography screening for lung cancer: a case-control and cohort validation study. Ann Intern Med 2012;157(4): 242–50.

16. Li K, Hüsing A, Sookthai D, et al. Selecting high-risk individuals for lung cancer screening: a prospective evaluation of existing risk models and eligibility criteria in the german EPIC cohort. Cancer Prev Res (Phila) 2015;8(9):777–85.

17. Ten Haaf K, Jeon J, Tammemägi MC, et al. Risk prediction models for selection of lung cancer screening candidates: a retrospective validation study. PLoS Med 2017;14(4):e1002277.

18. Weber M, Yap S, Goldsbury D, et al. Identifying high risk individuals for targeted lung cancer screening: Independent validation of the PLCO(m2012) risk prediction tool. Int J Cancer 2017;141(2):242–53.

19. Katki HA, Kovalchik SA, Petito LC, et al. Implications of nine risk prediction models for selecting ever-smokers for computed tomography lung cancer screening. Ann Intern Med 2018;169(1):10–9.

20. Robbins HA, Alcala K, Swerdlow AJ, et al. Comparative performance of lung cancer risk models to define lung screening eligibility in the United Kingdom. Br J Cancer 2021;124(12):2026–34.

21. Bhardwaj M, Schöttker B, Holleczek B, Brenner H. Comparison of discrimination performance of 11 lung cancer risk models for predicting lung cancer in a prospective cohort of screening-age adults from Germany followed over 17 years. Lung Cancer 2022;174:83–90.

22. Bach PB, Kattan MW, Thornquist MD, et al. Variations in lung cancer risk among smokers. J Natl Cancer Inst 2003;95(6):470–8.

23. Tammemägi MC, Katki HA, Hocking WG, et al. Selection criteria for lung-cancer screening. N Engl J Med 2013;368(8):728–36.

24. Katki HA, Kovalchik SA, Berg CD, Cheung LC, Chaturvedi AK. Development and validation of risk models to select ever-smokers for CT lung cancer screening. JAMA 2016;315(21):2300–11.

25. Cassidy A, Myles JP, van Tongeren M, et al. The LLP risk model: an individual risk prediction model for lung cancer. Br J Cancer 2008;98(2): 270–6.

26. Field JK, Duffy SW, Baldwin DR, et al. UK Lung Cancer RCT Pilot Screening Trial: baseline findings from the screening arm provide evidence for the potential implementation of lung cancer screening. Thorax 2016;71(2):161–70.

27. Crosbie PA, Gabe R, Simmonds I, et al. Yorkshire Lung Screening Trial (YLST): protocol for a randomised controlled trial to evaluate invitation to community-based low-dose CT screening for lung cancer versus usual care in a targeted population at risk,. BMJ Open 2020;10(9):e037075.

28. Lim KP, Marshall H, Tammemägi M, et al. Protocol and rationale for the international lung screening trial. Ann Am Thorac Soc 2020;17(4):503–12.

29. Pasquinelli MM, Tammemägi MC, Kovitz KL, et al. Risk prediction model versus United States Preventive Services Task Force 2020 draft lung cancer screening eligibility criteria-reducing race disparities. JTO Clin Res Rep 2021;2(3):100137.

30. Pasquinelli MM, Tammemägi MC, Kovitz KL, et al. Addressing sex disparities in lung cancer screening eligibility: USPSTF vs PLCOm2012 Criteria. Chest 2022;161(1):248–56.

31. Kumar V, Cohen JT, van Klaveren D, et al. Risk-targeted lung cancer screening: a cost-effectiveness analysis. Ann Intern Med 2018;168(3):161–9.

32. Cheung LC, Berg CD, Castle PE, Katki HA, Chaturvedi AK. Life-gained-based versus risk-based selection of smokers for lung cancer screening. Ann Intern Med 2019;171(9):623–32.

33. Toumazis I, Alagoz O, Leung A, Plevritis SK. A risk-based framework for assessing real-time lung cancer screening eligibility that incorporates life expectancy and past screening findings. Cancer 2021; 127(23):4432–46.

34. Caverly TJ, Cao P, Hayward RA, Meza R. Identifying patients for whom lung cancer screening is preference-sensitive: a microsimulation study. Ann Intern Med Jul 3 2018;169(1):1–9.

35. American College of Radiology. Available at: https://www.acr.org/Clinical-Resources/Reporting-and-Data-Systems/Lung-Rads. Accessed January 28, 2023.
36. Swensen SJ, Silverstein MD, Ilstrup DM, Schleck CD, Edell ES. The probability of malignancy in solitary pulmonary nodules. Application to small radiologically indeterminate nodules. Arch Intern Med 1997;157(8):849–55.
37. Gould MK, Ananth L, Barnett PG. A clinical model to estimate the pretest probability of lung cancer in patients with solitary pulmonary nodules. Chest 2007; 131(2):383–8.
38. Li Y, Chen KZ, Wang J. Development and validation of a clinical prediction model to estimate the probability of malignancy in solitary pulmonary nodules in Chinese people. Clin Lung Cancer 2011;12(5): 313–9.
39. McWilliams A, Tammemagi MC, Mayo JR, et al. Probability of cancer in pulmonary nodules detected on first screening CT. N Engl J Med 2013;369(10): 910–9.
40. Al-Ameri A, Malhotra P, Thygesen H, et al. Risk of malignancy in pulmonary nodules: a validation study of four prediction models. Lung Cancer 2015;89(1): 27–30.
41. Cui X, Heuvelmans MA, Han D, et al. Comparison of Veterans Affairs, Mayo, Brock classification models and radiologist diagnosis for classifying the malignancy of pulmonary nodules in Chinese clinical population. Transl Lung Cancer Res 2019;8(5):605–13.
42. Hammer MM, Nachiappan AC, Barbosa EJM Jr. Limited utility of pulmonary nodule risk calculators for managing large nodules. Curr Probl Diagn Radiol Jan-Feb 2018;47(1):23–7.
43. Talwar A, Rahman NM, Kadir T, Pickup LC, Gleeson F. A retrospective validation study of three models to estimate the probability of malignancy in patients with small pulmonary nodules from a tertiary oncology follow-up centre. Clin Radiol 2017;72(2): 177.e1–8.
44. Uthoff J, Koehn N, Larson J, et al. Post-imaging pulmonary nodule mathematical prediction models: are they clinically relevant? Eur Radiol 2019;29(10): 5367–77.
45. Vachani A, Zheng C, Amy Liu IL, Huang BZ, Osuji TA, Gould MK. The Probability of lung cancer in patients with incidentally detected pulmonary nodules: clinical characteristics and accuracy of prediction models. Chest 2022;161(2):562–71.
46. González Maldonado S, Delorme S, Hüsing A, et al. Evaluation of prediction models for identifying malignancy in pulmonary nodules detected via low-dose computed tomography. JAMA Netw Open 2020; 3(2):e1921221.
47. Kim H, Kim HY, Goo JM, Kim Y. External validation and comparison of the Brock model and Lung-RADS for the baseline lung cancer CT screening using data from the Korean Lung Cancer Screening Project. Eur Radiol. Jun 2021;31(6):4004–15.
48. van Riel SJ, Ciompi F, Jacobs C, et al. Malignancy risk estimation of screen-detected nodules at baseline CT: comparison of the PanCan model, Lung-RADS and NCCN guidelines. Eur Radiol 2017; 27(10):4019–29.
49. Maisonneuve P, Bagnardi V, Bellomi M, et al. Lung cancer risk prediction to select smokers for screening CT–a model based on the Italian COSMOS trial. Cancer Prev Res (Phila) 2011;4(11): 1778–89.
50. Veronesi G, Maisonneuve P, Rampinelli C, et al. Computed tomography screening for lung cancer: results of ten years of annual screening and validation of cosmos prediction model. Lung Cancer 2013; 82(3):426–30.
51. Tammemägi MC, Ten Haaf K, Toumazis I, et al. Development and validation of a multivariable lung cancer risk prediction model that includes low-dose computed tomography screening results: a secondary analysis of data from the national lung screening trial. JAMA Netw Open 2019;2(3): e190204.
52. Robbins HA, Cheung LC, Chaturvedi AK, Baldwin DR, Berg CD, Katki HA. Management of lung cancer screening results based on individual prediction of current and future lung cancer risks. J Thorac Oncol 2022;17(2):252–63.
53. Cressman S, Weber MF, Ngo PJ, et al. Economic impact of using risk models for eligibility selection to the International lung screening Trial. Lung Cancer 2022;176:38–45.
54. Tammemägi MC, Ruparel M, Tremblay A, et al. USPSTF2013 versus PLCOm2012 lung cancer screening eligibility criteria (International Lung Screening Trial): interim analysis of a prospective cohort study. Lancet Oncol 2022;23(1): 138–48.
55. Caverly TJ, Meza R. Using risk models to make lung cancer screening decisions: evidence-based and getting better. Ann Intern Med 2019;171(9):669–70.
56. Tammemägi MC, Church TR, Hocking WG, et al. Evaluation of the lung cancer risks at which to screen ever- and never-smokers: screening rules applied to the PLCO and NLST cohorts. PLoS Med 2014;11(12):e1001764.
57. Kerpel-Fronius A, Tammemägi M, Cavic M, et al. Screening for lung cancer in individuals who never smoked: an international association for the study of lung cancer early detection and screening committee report. J Thorac Oncol 2022;17(1):56–66.
58. Fukunaga MI, Halligan K, Kodela J, et al. Tools to promote shared decision-making in lung cancer screening using low-dose CT scanning: a systematic review. Chest 2020;158(6):2646–57.

59. Studts JL, Thurer RJ, Brinker K, Lillie SE, Byrne MM. Brief education and a conjoint valuation survey may reduce decisional conflict regarding lung cancer screening. MDM Policy Pract 2020;5(1). 2381468319891452.

60. Schapira MM, Chhatre S, Prigge JM, et al. A veteran-centric web-based decision aid for lung cancer screening: usability analysis. JMIR Form Res 2022; 6(4):e29039.

61. Lowery J, Fagerlin A, Larkin AR, Wiener RS, Skurla SE, Caverly TJ. Implementation of a web-based tool for shared decision-making in lung cancer screening: mixed methods quality improvement evaluation. JMIR Hum Factors 2022;9(2):e32399.

62. Kates FR, Romero R, Jones D, Egelfeld J, Datta S. A comparison of web-based cancer risk calculators that inform shared decision-making for lung cancer screening. J Gen Intern Med 2021;36(6):1543–52.

63. Sferra SR, Cheng JS, Boynton Z, et al. Aiding shared decision making in lung cancer screening: two decision tools. J Public Health (Oxf) 2021;43(3):673–80.

64. Hasan N, Kumar R, Kavuru MS. Lung cancer screening beyond low-dose computed tomography: the role of novel biomarkers. Lung 2014;192(5): 639–48.

65. Seijo LM, Peled N, Ajona D, et al. Biomarkers in Lung Cancer Screening: Achievements, Promises, and Challenges. J Thorac Oncol. 2019;14(3): 343–57.

66. Chapman CJ, Healey GF, Murray A, et al. EarlyCDT®-Lung test: improved clinical utility through additional autoantibody assays. Tumour Biol 2012; 33(5):1319–26.

67. Sullivan FM, Mair FS, Anderson W, et al. Earlier diagnosis of lung cancer in a randomised trial of an auto-antibody blood test followed by imaging. Eur Respir J 2021;57(1). https://doi.org/10.1183/13993003.00670-2020.

68. Doseeva V, Colpitts T, Gao G, Woodcock J, Knezevic V. Performance of a multiplexed dual analyte immunoassay for the early detection of non-small cell lung cancer. J Transl Med. Feb 12 2015; 13:55.

69. Nardi-Agmon I, Abud-Hawa M, Liran O, et al. Exhaled breath analysis for monitoring response to treatment in advanced lung cancer. J Thorac Oncol 2016;11(6):827–37.

70. Peled N, Hakim M, Bunn PA Jr, et al. Non-invasive breath analysis of pulmonary nodules. J Thorac Oncol 2012;7(10):1528–33.

71. Spira A, Beane JE, Shah V, et al. Airway epithelial gene expression in the diagnostic evaluation of smokers with suspect lung cancer. Nat Med 2007; 13(3):361–6.

72. Silvestri GA, Vachani A, Whitney D, et al. A bronchial genomic classifier for the diagnostic evaluation of lung cancer. N Engl J Med 2015;373(3):243–51.

73. Raval AA, Benn BS, Benzaquen S, et al. Reclassification of risk of malignancy with Percepta Genomic Sequencing Classifier following nondiagnostic bronchoscopy. Respir Med 2022;204:106990.

74. Sethi S, Oh S, Chen A, et al. Percepta genomic sequencing classifier and decision-making in patients with high-risk lung nodules: a decision impact study. BMC Pulm Med 2022;22(1):26.

75. Mathios D, Johansen JS, Cristiano S, et al. Detection and characterization of lung cancer using cell-free DNA fragmentomes. Nat Commun 2021;12(1):5060.

76. Montani F, Marzi MJ, Dezi F, et al. miR-Test: a blood test for lung cancer early detection. J Natl Cancer Inst 2015;107(6):djv063.

77. Sozzi G, Boeri M, Rossi M, et al. Clinical utility of a plasma-based miRNA signature classifier within computed tomography lung cancer screening: a correlative MILD trial study. J Clin Oncol 2014; 32(8):768–73.

78. Meyer MG, Hayenga JW, Neumann T, et al. The Cell-CT 3-dimensional cell imaging technology platform enables the detection of lung cancer using the noninvasive LuCED sputum test. Cancer Cytopathol 2015;123(9):512–23.

79. Hung RJ, Warkentin MT, Brhane Y, et al. Assessing lung cancer absolute risk trajectory based on a polygenic risk model. Cancer Res 2021;81(6):1607–15.

UNITED STATES POSTAL SERVICE ®

Statement of Ownership, Management, and Circulation (All Periodicals Publications Except Requester Publications)

1. Publication Title	2. Publication Number	3. Filing Date
THORACIC SURGERY CLINICS	013 – 126	9/18/2023

4. Issue Frequency	5. Number of Issues Published Annually	6. Annual Subscription Price
FEB, MAY, AUG, NOV	4	$417.00

7. Complete Mailing Address of Known Office of Publication (Not printer) (Street, city, county, state, and ZIP+4®)

ELSEVIER INC.
230 Park Avenue, Suite 800
New York, NY 10169

Contact Person
Malathi Samayan

Telephone (include area code)
91-44-4299-4507

8. Complete Mailing Address of Headquarters or General Business Office of Publisher (Not printer)

ELSEVIER INC.
230 Park Avenue, Suite 800
New York, NY 10169

9. Full Names and Complete Mailing Addresses of Publisher, Editor, and Managing Editor (Do not leave blank)

Publisher (Name and complete mailing address)

Dolores Meloni, ELSEVIER INC.
1600 JOHN F KENNEDY BLVD. SUITE 1600
PHILADELPHIA, PA 19103-2899

Editor (Name and complete mailing address)

JOHN VASSALLO, ELSEVIER INC.
1600 JOHN F KENNEDY BLVD. SUITE 1600
PHILADELPHIA, PA 19103-2899

Managing Editor (Name and complete mailing address)

PATRICK MANLEY, ELSEVIER INC.
1600 JOHN F KENNEDY BLVD. SUITE 1600
PHILADELPHIA, PA 19103-2899

10. Owner (Do not leave blank. If the publication is owned by a corporation, give the name and address of the corporation immediately followed by the names and addresses of all stockholders owning or holding 1 percent or more of the total amount of stock. If not owned by a corporation, give the names and addresses of the individual owners. If owned by a partnership or other unincorporated firm, give its name and address as well as those of each individual owner. If the publication is published by a nonprofit organization, give its name and address.)

Full Name	Complete Mailing Address
WHOLLY OWNED SUBSIDARY OF REED/ELSEVIER, US HOLDINGS	1600 JOHN F KENNEDY BLVD, SUITE 1600 PHILADELPHIA, PA 19103-2899

11. Known Bondholders, Mortgagees, and Other Security Holders Owning or Holding 1 Percent or More of Total Amount of Bonds, Mortgages, or Other Securities. If none, check box → ☐ None

Full Name	Complete Mailing Address
N/A	

12. Tax Status (For completion by nonprofit organizations authorized to mail at nonprofit rates) (Check one)
The purpose, function, and nonprofit status of this organization and the exempt status for federal income tax purposes:
☒ Has Not Changed During Preceding 12 Months
☐ Has Changed During Preceding 12 Months (Publisher must submit explanation of change with this statement)

PS Form 3526, July 2014 [Page 1 of 4 (see instructions page 4)]   PSN: 7530-01-000-9931   PRIVACY NOTICE: See our privacy policy on www.usps.com.

---

13. Publication Title		14. Issue Date for Circulation Data Below
THORACIC SURGERY CLINICS		AUGUST 2023

15. Extent and Nature of Circulation			Average No. Copies Each Issue During Preceding 12 Months	No. Copies of Single Issue Published Nearest to Filing Date
a. Total Number of Copies (Net press run)			150	147
b. Paid Circulation (By Mail and Outside the Mail)	(1)	Mailed Outside-County Paid Subscriptions Stated on PS Form 3541 (include paid distribution above nominal rate, advertiser's proof copies, and exchange copies)	84	84
	(2)	Mailed In-County Paid Subscriptions Stated on PS Form 3541 (Include paid distribution above nominal rate, advertiser's proof copies, and exchange copies)	0	0
	(3)	Paid Distribution Outside the Mails Including Sales Through Dealers and Carriers, Street Vendors, Counter Sales, and Other Paid Distribution Outside USPS®	52	51
	(4)	Paid Distribution by Other Classes of Mail Through the USPS (e.g., First-Class Mail®)	11	9
c. Total Paid Distribution (Sum of 15b (1), (2), (3), and (4))			147	144
d. Free or Nominal Rate Distribution (By Mail and Outside the Mail)	(1)	Free or Nominal Rate Outside-County Copies included on PS Form 3541	3	3
	(2)	Free or Nominal Rate In-County Copies Included on PS Form 3541	0	0
	(3)	Free or Nominal Rate Copies Mailed at Other Classes Through the USPS (e.g., First-Class Mail)	0	0
	(4)	Free or Nominal Rate Distribution Outside the Mail (Carriers or other means)	0	0
e. Total Free or Nominal Rate Distribution (Sum of 15d (1), (2), (3) and (4))			3	3
f. Total Distribution (Sum of 15c and 15e)			150	147
g. Copies not Distributed (See Instructions to Publishers #4 (page 43))			0	0
h. Total (Sum of 15f and g)			150	147
i. Percent Paid (15c divided by 15f times 100)			98%	97.96%

* If you are claiming electronic copies, go to line 16 on page 3. If you are not claiming electronic copies, skip to line 17 on page 3.

PS Form 3526, July 2014 (Page 2 of 4)

16. Electronic Copy Circulation	Average No. Copies Each Issue During Preceding 12 Months	No. Copies of Single Issue Published Nearest to Filing Date
a. Paid Electronic Copies ▶		
b. Total Paid Print Copies (Line 15c) + Paid Electronic Copies (Line 16a) ▶		
c. Total Print Distribution (Line 15f) + Paid Electronic Copies (Line 16a) ▶		
d. Percent Paid (Both Print & Electronic Copies) (16b divided by 16c × 100) ▶		

☒ I certify that 60% of all my distributed copies (electronic and print) are paid above a nominal price.

17. Publication of Statement of Ownership

☒ If the publication is a general publication, publication of this statement is required. Will be printed in the NOVEMBER 2023 issue of this publication.   ☐ Publication not required.

18. Signature and Title of Editor, Publisher, Business Manager, or Owner	Date
Malathi Samayan — Distribution Controller Malathi Samayan	9/18/2023

I certify that all information furnished on this form is true and complete. I understand that anyone who furnishes false or misleading information on this form or who omits material or information requested on the form may be subject to criminal sanctions (including fines and imprisonment) and/or civil sanctions (including civil penalties).

PS Form 3526, July 2014 (Page 3 of 4)   PRIVACY NOTICE: See our privacy policy on www.usps.com.

Moving?

Make sure your subscription moves with you!

To notify us of your new address, find your **Clinics Account Number** (located on your mailing label above your name), and contact customer service at:

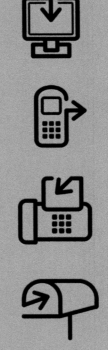

Email: journalscustomerservice-usa@elsevier.com

800-654-2452 (subscribers in the U.S. & Canada)
314-447-8871 (subscribers outside of the U.S. & Canada)

Fax number: 314-447-8029

Elsevier Health Sciences Division
Subscription Customer Service
3251 Riverport Lane
Maryland Heights, MO 63043

*To ensure uninterrupted delivery of your subscription, please notify us at least 4 weeks in advance of move.